3·50

A Description Concerning Such Mechanism as Will Afford a Nice, or True Mensuration of Time

A
DESCRIPTION
CONCERNING
SUCH MECHANISM
AS WILL AFFORD A NICE, OR TRUE
MENSURATION OF TIME, &c.

[Price THREE SHILLINGS fewed.]

A
DESCRIPTION

CONCERNING

SUCH MECHANISM

AS WILL AFFORD A NICE, OR TRUE

MENSURATION OF TIME;

TOGETHER WITH

SOME ACCOUNT

OF THE

ATTEMPTS for the DISCOVERY

OF THE

LONGITUDE BY THE MOON:

AS ALSO

AN ACCOUNT

OF THE

DISCOVERY

OF THE

SCALE OF MUSICK.

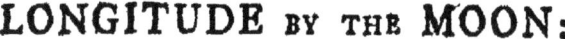

By JOHN HARRISON,

INVENTER of the TIME-KEEPER for the LONGITUDE
at SEA.

LONDON:
Printed for the AUTHOR, and fold by T. JONES,
No. 138, FETTER-LANE.

M.DCC LXXV.

―――――――――――――――――――――

Of the NATURE of a PENDULUM, as
primarily implying in itſelf; and
ſeſondarily, as when, according to
any particular Manner [good or
bad] in which it may be applied
to the Draught of the Wheels of
a Clock, &c.

AS firſt, or rather as here at the firſt,
[viz. as] without the taking any
Notice of the great or chief Matter, viz. of
what pertains to different Vibrations, or
rather, as more properly ſpeaking, of what
Advantage pertains to, or accrues from the
Largeneſs of a Vibration] the bare Length of
a Pendulum can be no otherwiſe rightly
conſidered or eſteemed, but as only to what
it bears, or may [as according to the common Application] bear in Proportion to the
Length of the Pallats, and as together with
ſuch improper Powers or Circumſtances
thereunto belonging, or may, as farther
thereunto belong; i. e. in other Words, [and
as ſtill in the firſt Place] to the equivalent

B   Diſtance

Diftance from its Center of Motion, to where the Pallats, (according to their Conftruction, and as may, or will continually happen with ~~their different States~~ of the Oil, as in the common Way) touch, or are applied to the Wheel ; nay, fometimes fome Men, ~~as being quite ignorant in what I am here about to fhew or fpeak of, and as when they are about to do fomething very extraordinary as they imagine,~~ do render the Matter ~~as~~ ftill worfe ~~then fo,~~ yea even by far ; ~~whenas the which,~~ as my good Friend Mr. Graham ordered the Matter, [~~viz.~~ in what are now called Aftronomical Clocks, notwithftanding their being but ftill, as an uncertain Sort of Regulators, or defective Time-keepers] the Pendulum, ~~as~~ with refpect to the Length of the Pallats, ~~and as here in the firft Place to be notified,~~ being no more than ~~as~~ ⌜about⌝ $14\frac{1}{2}$ to 1, ~~fo~~ the which in Effect is no better, or can in Power [~~as even in this Point the Length~~] be no better, than as a long Pendulum rendered a fhort one. And ~~whenas~~ farther, it is ~~withal~~ to be obferved, ~~viz. as~~ according to Mr. Graham's Method, [~~and as even already in fome Meafure intimated~~] that, as in the Time in which his Pendulum-Wheel is acting, fo as ~~whereby~~ to maintain the Motion, or ~~as here, to the Purpofe~~ more properly fpeaking, the poor, little, or feeble Motion of his Pendulum, that, I fay, as the fame is fo to be let, viz. through or from the great floping of the Pallats or Manner

of

of fcaping, fo as to jam, wedge, puſh or
prefs forward, viz. as with a much quicker
Motion, nay, as thence to be fuffered even
to pafs through twice fo much Space, as, in
during that Space of Time the Pallats, or
each Pallat has to recede or move from it,
[viz. from the Wheel, or as in Perpendicu-
lars thereto] and as when the ſame [or as
notwithſtanding the ſame] muſt, as moreover be in Effect, as ſtill a great ſhortening
or Diſadvantage to the Power or Regulation
of the Pendulum; for, upon a right Con-
ſideration, as when taken in with the other,
[viz. with the Length of the Pallats, or the
Diſtance of their Action from their reſpective
Center, or that of the Pendulum's Suſpenſion]
the Pendulum muſt, as thence in the whole,
be rendered as a very ſhort one indeed, yea,
fo ſhort [as with reſpect to the ſame Conſtruction of Pallats] as hardly to be eſteemed
fo much as 10 to 1; nay, [from what has
been ſhewn] it cannot be ſaid to be amifs, if
I ſay, but as $7\frac{1}{4}$ to 1; a very improper Proceeding fure! *   And that, as not only with
regard to the inconſtant Action, Dominion,

B 2   or

* And as here, by the by, a very bad Example for
Church and Turret Clocks, for in them [in this Diſpoſi-
tion of the Pallats, or Dead-beat-way, as according to
Mr. Graham] even the different Weight of the Rope,
viz. betwixt the Weight being up and almoſt down, will
greatly affect the Vibrations of the Pendulum, as alſo
the ſame in the diſcharging of the ſtriking part. Nay,
Mr. Graham himſelf did not think it to be proper, that
one

or Power of the Wheel or Wheels, by the
faid Pallats to the Pendulum, but as ~~more~~
~~efpecially, or as rather~~ on the other Hand,
~~by or~~ from the ill Confequence of fuch an
improper Conftruction of Pallats, ~~viz. as~~
with Regard to their communicating the
natural Stability or Regularity of the Pendulum to the Clock ; *i. e.* in the whole as in
other Words, and as without any Provifion
to the contrary, viz. fo as that no fuch Uncertainty as might ever happen, and 'as' in
the firft ~~or chief~~ Place from the faid Pallats
themfelves, or the Oil upon them, and that
as at their vaft Length from the Center of
Motion of the Pendulum as above ; neither,
as fecondly, from any Difference in the
Draught of the Wheels of the Clock, as from
the faid Oil at their Pevets, nor as elfewhere,
or otherwife to be occafioned, and ~~as~~ to be
by ~~fuch~~ the fame Pallats conveyed to, or
impreffed upon the Pendulum, fhould ever
be able to prevent or affect the Regularity of
the fame ; whenas there is nothing at all
towards thefe in the Matter ! but only as it
were, on the contrary, the bad Effects or
Embarraffment

---

one of his Clocks fhould fo much as have a Day of the
Month to fhift, [and well he might not] whenas,
to a right Application of the Pendulum, [and in fuppofing, as in common, all the Wheels concerned] that
muft be as nothing, was it to go harder than what it
needs to do ; and as with regard to Church and Turret
Clocks, there is Room for great Improvement, viz.
as in Comparifon to what is hitherto done.

Embarraffment [and in a bad Manner] of
more or lefs uncertain Friction! or of fuch
Differences as may or will continually happen
therein! viz. fuch as muft the moft efpecially
have a bad Influence upon fmall Vibrations,
as being fo nonfenfically coincident in the
Pallats, as at fo remote, or as even at fo
rudely remote a Diftance from the Center of
motion of the Pendulum! But as notwithftanding, the learned Part of the World
[through Mr. Graham] is become fo ftu-
pidly confident in the Nonfenfe, as hardly
to be perfuaded that any Thing elfe can
ever be better; they indeed, [viz. the
Public] not having as yet [as I have] any
Experience to the contrary; nor hitherto
has right Steps been taken ever for them to
have it; but that they might ftill keep in
the Dark, or at leaft in a Mift as they have
done; whenas, it has ever been furprifing
to me, how fuch Stupidity could take Place,
and fpread itfelf in the World; for the firft
Time I faw Mr. Graham, and he fhewed it
me, I thought, that either he muft be out of
his Senfes, or I muft be fo! Now, as
touching the Matter, or firft Matter in mine,
viz. the Length of the Pendulum, as with
refpect to the Diftance from its Center of
Motion, to where the Force of the Wheel is
applied, is about in Proportion as 100 to 1,
and as without any fuch wedge-like thrufting as fpoken of above, and as withal with
no different Clamminefs of Oil, there not

being,

being, from the Conſtruction and Material of my Pallats, any Oil required, but as on the other Hand, and as implying, at a ſmall Diſtance from the Center of Motion of the Pendulum, and that beſides ſuch other ~~Virtue or~~ Virtues as below, the Friction at the ſaid Pallats to be ſo far diminiſhed by the Contrivance, as not to come to the 100ᵉᵈ. Part of what is in the common Way, no, not when in ~~that Way [as meaning the ſame in~~ Mr. Graham's Way] the Oil is in its greateſt State of Fluidity ; but, indeed, ~~as~~ with reſpect to ~~this latter Article, viz.~~ the very ſmall Quantity of Friction at the Pallats, it in itſelf may be eſteemed, ~~as~~ with reſpect to the Length of the Pendulum, to where its Effect is from the Center of Motion of the Pendulum, to be but as about 44 to 1, but ſtill, ~~as whence~~ from its Smallneſs, as juſt above ſpoken of, it muſt be rendered ſo as to become in Effect ~~even as~~ quite inſenſible, immaterial or nothing, ~~nay, as not in the whole, when rightly conſidered, to be worth any notifying at all~~ ; and ~~withal~~, as the Pevets of the Arbor of the Pallats and Crouch are made of Braſs, and are only as Edges of a very acute Angle, and move in poliſhed Notches cut in Glaſs, ſo the Friction there muſt alſo be inſenſible ; for, if ~~for an Example in this Point,~~ the ſaid Crouch [or Communicator of the Force of the Wheel, by the Pallats to the Pendulum, and as for this Experiment, without the Pendulum upon a Table] be ſet to vibrate

vibrate only fo far, as not to caufe the Pallats
to touch or be concerned with the Wheel,
it will be 10 Minutes before it comes to
reft, the which the Air [at the Rate it will
vibrate with its Returns, and as fo light a
Matter] may be fuppofed fufficient in that
Space of Time to occafion. But it is alledged,
in Mr. Graham's Cafe, [viz. in the Wheel's
acting upon the Pendulum] at fo far a
Diftance from the Center of Motion of the
Pendulum] that a much lefs Force, or a very
fmall Force from the Wheel, will keep the
Pendulum in Motion ; an idle Way, indeed,
to confider the Thing ¹ fince [and even as
already implied] it is not properly [or fin-
gularly] Force from the Wheel that can occafion a Variation in the Motion of the Pendulum, for the bigger the Force the Wheel
can well or rightly be permitted to have,
the more conftant or certain that Force will
be to itfelf; fo from (the Point in Hand) or
from fo far as belongs to it, * any Variation
in the Menfuration of Time, muft, as above,
be from the different States of the Oil, and
as chiefly at the Pallats, viz. as with regard
to the Smallnefs of the Force from the Wheel

[fince

---

* A firm Sufpenfion of the Pendulum to be, as in the
firft Place, made fure of, viz. from a firm Wall, as not
having, or to have any Dependance from the Clock, the
Clock-Cafe, or any Wainfcot; for as without that, and
as hitherto in common, all muft be no better than
Chance, as with refpect to any true Performance of a
clock.

[fince Differences therein will be the greater in Proportion] and as when the fame is ~~withal~~ to be taken or confidered at the Greatnefs of the Diftance from the Center of Motion of the Pendulum, to where it is [as with fuch Differences] applied by the Pallats thereto. and as ftill together with the coherent, or ~~rather~~ coincident Smallnefs, Weaknefs, or Feeblenefs in the Vibration, there muft, I fay, Variations arife from the whole ; for, ~~as farther~~, was it to be better for a fmall Force from the Wheel to maintain the Motion of the Pendulum, it would then be the beft for the Wheel to act at fuch a Length of Pallats as to be equivalent to that of the Pendulum, for then [and as withal to be with or for fuch an infignificant Vibration, as could but hardly be faid to be a Vibration, but ftill fuch as muft be coincident in the Matter] a very minutely Force would do; but, I pray, to what Purpofe? for where would then be the Property or Power of a Pendulum at all, viz. as with Regard to fuch Inftability as muft or would attend fuch a Force, [could, as moft unreafonably, the fame be always fuppofed to exift] and as even in fuppofing the Bob to be immenfely heavy? [And yet to this Mr. Graham's Product is pretty much a-kin, or at leaft bears thereunto too great a Proportion !] And ~~as~~ therefore ~~from whence, as~~ by Way of Corollary, ~~and as a Tenor~~ to be extended to all that can be faid of this Point in general, that through
the

the Pendulum Wheel's paffing by any Means,
as [if you pleafe] in unregarded Proportion,
or as in any Proportion through too much
Space in a Second, [or Piece of a Second] and
the Pendulum through too little, [viz. in
each of its Swings] muft give the Wheel and
Pallats, with what may attend them, too
much Mafterfhip over, or bad Effect upon
the Pendulum; infomuch, that the different
States of the Oil, and as chiefly at the Pallats, and as together, and as partly thereby
occafioned from the different States of the
Air, both muft and will occafion confiderable
Variations in the Motion of the Clock; for
as when from either of thefe, or any Càufe
whatever, Friction at the Pallats is increafed,
a Touch of frefh Oil thereunto applied, [viz.
at one or two of the Teeth of the Pendulum-
Wheel] I mean, whether in Mr. Graham's
way, as now very common, or whether in
the other, as yet, or ftill the more common,
will occafion a different Motion of the Pendulum; but, as in Mr. Graham's Way,
through the very great or improper floping,
or as it were wedge-like thrufting, or jamming Scapement of the Pallats, viz. fo as
whereby to fuffer the Wheel to move or pafs
much fafter forward, than each Pallat as at
right Angles has to recede from it, and at fo
great a Diftance from the Center of Motion
of the Pendulum, and as together with the
coherent Weaknefs or Feeblenefs of the Motion thereof, and that as through the Smallnefs

nefs of its Vibration or Arch it defcribes, [O he] and as moft efpecially fo, when the Clock or its Oil grows foul, the Touch of Oil (as here above-mentioned) will occafion the Pendulum to fetch a greater Arch, and the Clock thereby to go the fafter, [O he, I fay!] as was (according to my Reafon for the Matter) occafionally experienced and teftified by Dr. Bradley, for from which he found [as at the Juncture, Seafon, or as upon the occafion he did it] a Variation or Alteration in its Motion of about 2 Seconds a Day fafter; and had the Pevets of the Wheels been alfo (as at the fame Time) touched with Oil, it would doubtlefs-then-have gone fafter ftill; * whenas the fame Touch or Touches of Oil, as upon Occafion applied to the other Way, viz. where the Vibrations are larger, will

* Now it is to be notified, that as Mr. Graham had not the Redoublings of his Brafs and Steel Wires [viz. as in my Invention of the Compound Pendulum] fo long by a good deal, no, not even by 2 Inches or more, than as what I had found to be required therein, [for, as otherwife, my Clock would go too flow in Summer] whence it muft be plain, or as a Proof to the Matter, that from the extravagant Length of Pallats he ufed, viz. as acting upon the Pendulum at fo great a Diftance from the Center of Motion of the Pendulum, and as together with their powerful floping, pufhing, jamming or wedging; and when, as farther, in or for fuch little or feeble Vibrations thereof, as thence to be defcribed, muft have, as generally fpeaking when warm, a greater Power through Glibnefs, to haften fuch the faid feeble or fmall Vibrations of the Pendulum, [the Pendulum being then, had Matters been right, as here above to be underftood, too

will (as above) make the Pendulum to fetch the farther, but the Clock thereby to go the flower, the which muft be, nay, is in this Point the better, becaufe as ~~here [or as~~ in this latter Cafe] it is according to the Nature of the Pendulum, whenas it is plain, that ~~as~~ in the other, it proves the Contrivance to be ~~even as~~ quite contradictory to it, meer ~~Corruption~~ ! yea, ~~as~~ notwithftanding any fuch Maffinefs as may or ever can be in the Bob, viz. ~~as~~ with refpect to the Force that is to maintain its Motion ! * confequently, was there no other Matter or Matters in the Affair but this, whenas, to come to the Truth, ~~or to a continuing Truth~~, there are other Things befides this, and they of very great
Moment ;

too long] than as when from that, their improper Principle, to be attended with Clamminefs when cold [I fay this muft be the Cafe, as generally fpeaking] and to which the Refult of Dr. Bradley's touching his Pendulum-Wheel with Oil, agrees exactly well, it being to be underftood, viz. from what is here above as firft advanced in this Note, that the fhorter the Redoublings of the Wires, the longer the Pendulum when warm.

* And upon this Head it may, or is to be notified, that fome have fpoke of how long a Pendulum will vibrate when exempt from the Wheels of a Clock, as taking no Notice of how long it will vibrate when at a Clock, and as when fet at fo low a Vibration, as not to fuffer the Pallats to interchange, but as when the Force or Action of the Pendulum-Wheel is to lean againft one of the Pallats, or long Pallats, for during the Time of that Experiment, neither any Notice of the moft chief, viz. of the Difference there will be (in that Cafe) betwixt when the Pallats and Wheel are clean and new oiled, to what there will be when foul.

Moment; but I fay, as in Confequence to the Matter here, and as with the Pallats fhorter, and the Wheel with a Draught fuitably bigger, a Propernefs, viz. as when, as thence from Experience in the Largenefs of the Pendulum's Vibrations, and as with a proper recoiling of the Wheel inftead of lying dead ought to have been acquired, and not to have let or occafioned fo many Things to be made as upon fo very improper, ~~or as it were degenerated~~ Principle ; * but ftill, though it might have come ~~pretty~~ much ~~nearer, as according to what I have illuftrated, viz. as thence~~ nearer to the Truth in

---

* Now it is, or muft be very proper, that this fhould be put into Writing, left at any Time, or as ftill hereafter, even fo much as 2 Seconds a Day, as in Mr. Graham's Clocks, at diftant Times may or will fometimes, or rather often times happen, from natural Caufes, [viz. *as in fuppofing the Nut of the Pendulum Screw to be let to remain untouched, or unhitched, after it is once fuppofed, or the Clock fuppofed, or taken to be as truly adjufted*] I fay it muft be proper, left fuch a Matter fhould never be thought to be rightly accounted for, as here above I am very fure it is ; but had he, and as even with the fame prepofterous Length of Pallats he ufed, fo ordered the Matter, as that the floping of the faid Pallats, viz. as in the Manner he did it, [and as intimated, at fuch an enormous, extravagant, or unreafonable Diftance from the Center of Motion of the Pendulum] was not to have been fuffered to begin its Action upon the Pendulum (viz. as from the Wheel) till fome Time after, or paft the Middle of each Vibration, viz. fo much after as perhaps about one 6th part of fuch a Vibration, [or of fuch his fmall Vibration] or perhaps [as Differences muft continually happen therein] fomewhat more or lefs, but as beft to have been acquired

in general, yet ſtill, ~~as I may make bold to~~
~~ſay, that~~ if any Oil be requiſed at the Pallats, [viz. in ſuch Pallats, Caſe or Caſes, as I
am here ſpeaking of] it will but hardly let
the

acquired from Experience, viz. ſo far as that might have
been able to do it, as not meaning as thence, or from its
Nature, ever in anywiſe to have been done to Perfection,
and as when meaning withal, the Pendulum to be firm-
ly ſuſpended with Braſs or Iron from the Wall , for, as
without which, it could but be as a very ſhort or deficient Progreſs , but as then, viz. as from a more proper
Beginning of the Action of the Pallats upon the Pendulum, the Caſe as much for the better might have been
different, and that, as not only with Reſpect to the Touch
of Oil at the Pallats, [or, as above, Pendulum-Wheel]
but as alſo with Reſpect to a different Force from the
Wheels , for here I muſt let it to be underſtood, that the
later any Help or Force in any Vibration is given, [viz.
for the Maintenances thereof] the longer Time it will
take up in its being performed ; and as thence withal,
[or as in Conſequence] the greater that Force [or rather
Pop, as I may here, viz. as in Mr. Graham's Caſe, term
it] the longer each Vibration will, or would as thence
ſtill be, viz. as jointly by or from its Lateneſs, or, as
mathematically ſpeaking, the more Time each muſt as
ſtill take up in its being performed ; conſequently Glib-
neſs here might not occaſion the Clock to go faſter, but
might as eaſily make it go ſlower, the Matter [as under
ſuch Circumſtances as above ſhewn] not being as a
Thing exactly to be nicked . but here as withal, this
muſt be with ſuppoſing the Contrivance to admit of ſuch
Lateneſs of the Pop, whenas it could not well do that,
becauſe of ſuch Length of Weakneſs that would as thence
be required at the Ends or Extremities of the Teeth of the
Pendulum-Wheel ; no, neither would that be all, but
that the Clock would as thence, viz from the Lateneſs
of the Pop, and as with the Littleneſs of the Vibration,
and Inſtability of the Force or Draught of the Pendulum-
Wheel, viz. as from its Smallneſs, be ſooner in Danger of
ſtanding ;

the Clock to go, as strictly speaking, two
Days alike, viz. as when the State of the
Weather is pretty much varying; nay, neither as in Mr. Graham's Way, nor as in the
other

standing; therefore, in the whole, a very deficient Proceeding, and one would even wonder, that among all
our Mathematicians and Geometricians, that any Thing
material should, for so long a Time, or for any Length
of Time, be pretended by it. I say, it ought at least,
as with regard to their Honour, to be taken as a Wonder
that they have not as yet seen this, viz. the Nonsense of
Over-sight in the Matter, and that as in the following
Light, where even Dr. Bradley's Touch of Oil, as under
the improper Circumstances as above shewn,, [viz. of so
small or feeble a Vibration, and as to be maintained by a
sudden, but as still with respect to the Matter, by such
a powerful Impulse or Pop, viz. as at so great a Distance
from the Center of Motion of the Pendulum] has not as
yet fairly unveiled to them the Weakness of the Matter,
must (I say) be short indeed, viz. so as that instead of a
lying dead, there ought (as in the improper Case) to be,
or to have been a little hooking,, or, as more properly
speaking, a little convexical slanting or bowing in that
same Part of the Pallats the other Way, in order [as in
some Measure] towards helping up the last Part of each
Vibration of the Pendulum, viz. in its Ascents, and the
same to hinder it in the Beginning of each of its De-
scents, [the Teeth of the Wheel being so to be curved
forward as to admit of that,—bad to execute] but from
whence in the whole, (though undiscovered by such
learned Men as above) the Clock to have gone somewhat
slower, [but that to be, or to have been taken in, in the
common adjusting] and not, as thence, faster by a Touch
of Oil; but this indeed where, or as together with so
much Friction or Difference therein, as here above at-
tending, would be a very uncertain Matter, viz in what
Portion it might want to be done, or could be rightly
done, and the redoubling of the Wires [viz. the Pro-
vision for Heat and Cold] would require to be longer,

as

other more common, even whether any Oil
was required at the Pallats or not, as the
Weather is variable, it or they would not
continue as quite the fame, viz. as with refpect to their action upon the Pendulum,
and certainly Mr. Graham's could not in
that Cafe have the Odds of the other, confequently the Wires, or the Compound of
the Pendulum for Heat and Cold, never as
thence to be truly adjufted, viz. as by or
from any Provifion whatever thereto, and
fo, as even in Confequence of that, [was
there nothing elfe] never to be rightly fit
for Aftronomy. But as here to defift from
treating of fuch Pallats as thofe, viz. as
where Oil muft be concerned, and not as
only fo, but as alfo [as hath been fhewn]
from fuch Imperfections as otherwife at-
tending, [and as from Mr. Graham received
in the World] it is to be underftood as followeth, viz. That in my Contrivance or
Conftruction of Pallats, no oiling [at the
fame] could ever occafion the Vibrations of
the Pendulum to alter, but, as on the other
Hand, would occafion fuch Mifchief at the
faid

as alfo the fame from the Latenefs of the Pop, as here
above, as may be gathered from what I have fhewn in
the Note laft above. But now as hence, or as from *p. 12.*
thefe affirmative Suppofals, [and that as the chief Matter
aimed at] is fairly fhewn the Impropernefs, or rather
the Impracticability, of a fmall Vibration, viz. as for
any certain Good or Truth, as the fame of which I
have as otherwife fhewn, and fhall as hereafter farther
fhew.

said Pallats, as not to fuffer them to interchange at all, confequently the Clock not to
go at all; but, as without that, they will
~~as~~ not only at all Times go, [viz. ~~as~~ in, all
Seafons] but that with fo great a Freedom
from Friction, as whence with fuch their o-
ther Properties or Qualifications ~~as~~ of which
hereafter, [and as being ~~withal~~ upon a far
more proper Foundation, viz. as touching
the whole Clock, than any heretofore] fo
that indeed a very great Truth, viz. as to lefs
than a Second in a Month, is as thence af-
certained; and it is certain that my next
Clock, when finifhed, properly fet up, and
duly adjufted, will come to the Truth nearer
ftill. And now if ~~this, or~~ any Part of this,
fhould be thought ftrange, ~~as~~ touching my
Friend Mr. Graham's Proceedings, then ~~(as~~
~~in fome Meafure parallel thereto) I may afk~~
~~the Reafon, why, out of fo many Hundreds~~
~~of Muficians as there are, and have been in~~
~~the World, [and fome of them alfo Mathe-~~
~~maticians] why, I fay, that no one had ever~~
~~as yet before difcovered the true or real Scale~~
~~of Mufic, or its Foundation? as of which~~
~~hereafter; but towards the Matter, as they~~
~~thought it to be, [or that it muft be] was~~
~~always an Acting in fome Meafure contrary,~~
~~and that as not to be taken in a fmall Degree,~~
~~contrary, I fay, to the Nature of the Thing,~~
~~viz. in tuning the Organ, Harpfichord,~~
~~and Spinnet? Nay, the great Mr. Handel~~
~~had his Organ, &c. fo tuned!~~ But as notwithftanding

~~withstanding, if it should still~~ be thought ~~strange~~ as with respect to my worthy Friend Mr. ~~Graham,~~ I will here certify, and ~~that~~ was it upon Oath, [~~as according to Lord Morton's Proceeding~~] that I neither have said, nor shall express, any Thing more than what, or as according to the Tenor of which I expressed by Times to Mr. Graham himself, Face to Face, as I may say, for we reasoned the Cases, or upon the Principles, more than once; nay once, and that in a very extraordinary Manner, was at the very first Time I saw him, and our reasoning, or as it were sometimes debating, [~~but still, as the main,~~ understanding ~~one another~~ very ~~well~~] ~~then~~ held from about Ten o'Clock in the Forenoon, 'till about Eight at Night, the Time which Dinner took up included, ~~for he invited me to stay~~ to dine, &c. Now it is ~~to be understood,~~ that I had along with me (as ~~affording the Principles upon which we reasoned) the Descriptions, with some Drawings of the principal Parts of the Pendulum Clock which I had made, and as also of them of my then intended Time-Keeper for the Longitude at Sea.~~ But here ~~it must be highly worth remarking, that~~ I at first made Application to Dr. Halley, and as he had long been observing for the Longitude by the Moon, and ~~as~~ then becoming quite tired of it, or thoroughly satisfied, ~~as~~ touching the Impossibility of its ever doing any certain Good, [but not then

C   so

so to be let known to me, but was afterwards told it me by Mr. Graham] received
me the better; and in his finding what I
came about to be as principally touching a
true Mensuration of Time, viz. for that
Purpose of Longitude; but as previous
thereto, viz. as in his finding my Dealings
with the Pendulum for a true Mensuration
of Time, to be very much contrary to Mr.
Graham's Thoughts of, or Proceedings in
the Matter, advised me therefore to go to
Mr. Graham, but that Advice went hard
with me, for I thought it as a Step very improper to be taken; but he told me, that in
the Way which I was in, viz. as by Ma-
chinery [for the Longitude] more than
Astronomy, that I should certainly be sent
to Mr. Graham, and therefore advised me to
go without any farther to do; certifying
me also, that Mr. Graham was a very honest
Man, and would do me no harm, viz. as by
pirating any Thing from me, but that on
the contrary, would certainly do me Good if
it was in his Power; but withal, cautioned
me how to begin with Mr. Graham, viz.
so as in as few Words as possible, to let him
to understand, that I had indeed something
worthy Notice to communicate to him; but
as notwithstanding that Piece of Advice,
and my doing my best as pursuant thereto,
Mr. Graham began, as I thought it, very
roughly with me, and the which had like
to have occasioned me to become rough too;
but

but however, we got the Ice broke, the which would not bear, and the Paſſage over was as I have ſhewn, and indeed he became as at laſt vaſtly ſurpriſed at the Thoughts or Methods I had taken, or had found Occaſion to take, and as thence found Reaſon enough to believe that my Clock might go to a Second in a Month, and that as in Conſequence to be, as in the firſt Place, of great Service in the adjuſting a Time-Keeper for the Longitude; and indeed, as according to Dr. Halley, Mr. Graham proved a very great Friend to me, viz. not only as by his Aſſiſtance at the Board of Longitude, &c. but alſo in his ſo willingly lending me Money, as without any Security or Intereſt, and by the which, together with what other Gentlemen were pleaſed to give me, I was encouraged; as Charles Stanhope, Eſq; 8ol. [viz. 2ol. a Time, at four different Times at which he came to ſee me, with my good and worthy Friend Mr. Folkes along with him] the Eaſt India Company 1ool. and ſeveral others who worthily contributed to my Expence, and ſtill Mr. Graham among the reſt, nay, as at one Time Mr. Graham, Mr. Folkes, Dr. Heberden, and Mr. Short, each 10 Guineas, Lord Barrington 5, and 10 from an unknown Hand. Now by theſe, with ſeveral others, [nay indeed a many others] I was encouraged, for otherwiſe, as from the Encouragement of the Public alone, I

could

could never have gone through what I did, go, nor confequently ever have made a Completion of the Matter. So now after this (as in fome Meafure hiftorical Piece) to proceed.

And firft, as letting the proper Circum- ftances, Quality, or Efficacy of the Pallats for a Pendulum as above treated of, and as when together with fuch their other un- parallelled Properties as below, to be fairly ot rightly confidered, it muft as in Confe- quence, and that as here in the firft Place follow, [viz. as from the Conftruction of the faid Pallats, and Diftance inverfely from the Center of Motion of the Pendu- lum, to where the Force or Draught of the Pendulum-Wheel is by them communi- cated to the faid Pendulum] that the Power a Pendulum muft as thence have, fo as whereby to regulate a Clock, muft, I fay, as in fuppofing the Bob of a certain Weight, be about as the Square of the Arch it defcribes ; therefore, as by Corol- lary, it muft then follow, that if a Bob of 3 Pounds Weight be fufficient to regulate a Clock, when the Pendulum defcribes an Arch of 12 Degrees, 48 Pounds muft be required to do the fame Execution, or to be the fame in Power, whereby to regulate, if the Pendulum defcribes but 3 Degrees ; but it is to be remembered, that this muft be as already implied, viz. as in fuppofing a proper Conftruction, or due Qualification

of

of Pallats, ftill, or as in both Cafes to be
applied, ~~whenas~~ the which, to fo fmall a
Vibration as in the latter, could not be, nor
does it want to be, neither was the which
in either, or ~~as~~ in any Cafe, ever done before mine, nor as yet right by any but me
no Model thereof, Draught, or fufficient
Inftruction being as yet communicated to
the World ; and as without which, although as it were my natural Road, would
ftill prove a very tedious Matter to others,
it being (as it were) fo very much out of
their beaten Path ; as indeed the Execution
of which [with what muft at firft pertain
thereto, and as without Inftruction] would,
or muft have been no eafy Matter to Mr.
Graham, was he to have fet about it, or was
his Integrity fo to have permitted him ;
but ftill, as with refpect to the Matter, Mr.
Graham faid to feveral Gentlemen, that for
my Improvement in Clock-Work, I de-
ferved 2000ol.—was no Longitude to be
concerned, and that becaufe, as he found
good Reafon to think, viz. that fuch Perfection by any other or others would never
have been, there being indeed a great deal
of Reafon, viz. as touching the whole Clock,
to fuppofe as he did on the contrary ; but
however, the Way or Ways they are in
will, or may do for common Ufes, but
can never do rightly for Aftronomy.

And now, as granting a large Vibration
to be neceffary, it farther remains to be
underftood,

underftood, that a Pendulum cannot ftill
truly or ftrictly regulate a Clock, viz. to
any continuing Perfection, nor could any
Thing of or as in lieu of what is called a
Cycloid, occafion it fo to do; unlefs, as
in the firft Place, the Force from the Wheel
whereby its Motion is to be maintained
againft the Air's Refiftance, be the very
fame, or can prove the very fame as with
refpect to it in the whole, as that its Vibrations, or [as here to fpeak more clofely
to my Conftruction of the Pallats] any two
of its Vibrations as next in Succeffion, *
may be performed exactly, or, as it were
mathematically fpeaking, in the fame Time
as if at the fame mathematical Length it
went, or as might be fuppofed it would go
by itfelf, [viz. as without any Force from
the Wheels of a Clock] in Vacuo; or at
leaft as nearly thereto as poffible in the Cafe,
or as to be conceived of the Matter, and
that as with ftill retaining the above-mentioned Qualities of the Pallats, for any De-
vice

---

* For it may be notified, as juft here hinted, that
the Actions of each Pallat are not equally the fame upon
the Pendulum, but not fo, as to be eafily perceived to
be otherwife, viz. as in the looking at the Clock, or
Seconds in Motion, although in this moft highly material Circumftance, or Conftruction of the Pallats,
pretty much different, but ftill, not fo to be taken [viz.
as with refpect to th effential Point here in Hand] as to
be any the leaft worfe for the fame, but as that the
Action of one with that of the other, are quite right,
for or to the Purpofe, as farther of which below.

vice in the fame to render it ; as the which,
from due Contemplation and Experience,
I perfected. For, as to this weighty Article, it is to be underftood, viz. from the
Conftruction of my Pallats, (as intimated
above) that the Force of my Pendulum-
Wheel is fo difpofed of, as that, whether
the faid Force at any Time becomes fomewhat greater or lefs in itfelf, or that the Air
at any Time gives fomewhat more or lefs
Refiftance to the Pendulum, or both, [fee
the Note] * it is the fame to it as here above
required,

* Now this highly material Matter is from the
Wheel's acting [by my Contrivance of the Pallats] more
weakly upon the Pendulum in each or every one of its
Defcents, viz. from the Extremity of each Vibration,
[and there, as at the firft, the weakeft of all] to the
Bottom or Middle of each, and then [as ftill conti-
nuing] more and more ftrongly upon the Pendulum in
each of its Afcents, and the ftrongeft of all juft before
the interchanging of the Pallats, and the which Interchanging not being, or to be far from the Extremity of
each Vibration, and in which little, or as it were overplus Part, a neceffary recoiling of the Wheel to be, viz.
as not only for the interchanging of the Pallats, the
which, as according to my Conftruction of the fame is
required, but as withal to have in fome Meafure to do
with the Effect of a Cycloid, but not to be the whole
Concern in that Matter , the Pendulum withal requiring to be [viz as from my Contrivance of its Combina-
tion of Brafs and Steel Wires] rather, as mathematically
fpeaking, fhorter when warm than when cold. But
as here, to come a little nearer in this material Point,
let, as I order the Matter; the Force [from the Wheel]
upon the Pendulum, as juft before the interchanging of
the Pallats, to be as by or from them the faid Pallats
fuppofed or taken as 3, then, as juft after their interchanging

required, [but indeed this muſt be with
ſuppoſing, as in the Note, or as with taking
for

changing, [and the Force to contrary Direction, it muſt
but be about as 2, that is, it muſt be ſo ordered, [as
may hereafter be obſerved by the Drawing] viz. as
that it be ſo by the taking, or ſuppoſing for the Purpoſe,
a Mean betwixt the Actions of each Pallat, and withal,
as farther to the Purpoſe, that, as in the little recoiling
of the Wheel, to become leſs and leſs to the Extremity
of each Vibration, but as whence, or as ſtill on Courſe,
the greater at any Time the whole Vibration may be,
of more Efficacy the ſame ſmall Force [and ſtill as it
were in the little recoiling] muſt from its Quantity or
Duration prove, and that in ſuch ſmall Meaſure as required, the reſters of the Pallats [viz. their Compoſers
to relative Reſt] having withal for the better a little to
do in the Matter, and the which is ſtill from, or as with
Reſpect to the Length or Shortneſs of the Time [though
always to be eſteemed as but little] that is to be occu-
pied in the recoiling, it being to be underſtood, that
was the Force of the ſaid Wheel, or Pendulum-Wheel,
to be diſpoſed of uniformly upon the Pendulum,
throughout the whole of each Vibration, that then the
bigger that Force, and as with ſome recoiling of the
Wheel, the more it muſt tend towards occaſioning a
greater Vibration, or ſomewhat a greater Vibration of
the Pendulum to be the ſooner performed, but that is
not the Caſe in what is, as juſt here above ſhewn, but,
to the Purpoſe, is otherwiſe to be taken or conſidered ;
as that the bigger the Force towards the latter End of
any Vibration, viz as in Compariſon to what it may be
at the fore End or Beginning, and as in ſuppoſing without a Recoil of the Wheel, the ſlower the Vibration
muſt be, or the longer the Time it muſt take up, as
mathematically ſpeaking, wherein to be performed, but
as with a proper recoiling, and artificial Cycloid,
rightly adapted, not ſo, viz. as when in ſuch Largeneſs
of Vibration as muſt to this Purpoſe, as well as to other
Purpoſes, be as the moſt neceſſarily herein required, and
as when, as muſt unavoidably be the Caſe, in the
moving

for granted, that the Pendulum muſt be
rather ſhorter when warm than when cold]
and

moving by the Draught of a Wheel, or of the Wheels
of a Clock in the Medium of Air, neither, as by any
Means, does a ſuitable Matter of this, viz. of the Air's
Reſiſtance, want to be avoided, as many have fooliſhly
imagined, but is of real or great Uſe, as the which I
ſhall ſhew preſently, and ſo, as I may make bold to
ſay, there has not as heretofore appeared in the World,
or to the Public, any Thing towards a ſtrict, or rather,
as along with other Things of mine, to, as I may ſay,
the moſt ſtrict or exact Menſuration of Time, and
where they muſt find any other Thing or Things equivalent, as according to Mr. Maſkelyne, viz equivalent
to my Clock here, or to my Watch as hereafter, I do
not know, nay, there is ſubſtantial Reaſon to think,
that that will never be known, no, although as without
Reaſon they ſhould ſtill make a many more Trials.
But to return, I have above in this Note, viz. as in a
Parentheſis ſaid, as may hereafter be obſerved by the
Drawing, i e. not meaning the Drawing and its Ex-
planation to be along with this Writing, my Encouragement not having ſuited, or, as in other Words, my
Reward for the Watch being too backward, ſo there
cannot well be an Obligation for that at preſent, altho'
it be the firſt Step; for I was only, and unreaſonably,
compelled to explain the Watch, viz. ſo far as I had
then advanced therein, and thought as concerning its
principal Parts, but indeed at that Time [though I told
them what I thought] there was as on my Behalf, ſome
Miſtakes [or not right Underſtanding] as touching
ſome of the Contrivances in the ſame, and here it may,
or is to be notified, that from no Experience of any Sea
Trial [viz as in my Way to work] is or was any Improvement ever to be made, no, ſuch Trials [or Sea
Trials] as with reſpect to what I have done, or had
then ſo far perfected, could only be as a Loſs of Time,
or Hindrance to the Matter [ſave only as once, in
order to fulfil the Letter of the Act of Parliament] but,
as notwithſtanding, through unſkilful, intereſted No-
viçes

and fo by Means of fomething at the Top,
but not according to Mr. Huygens's Demonftration

vices, viz. as put in Power, and though at the fame
Time learned Men, [ftiled Reverend] great Trouble
and Hinderance, and as attended with great Expence,
has that Way been occafion-
ed, ‖ they not wanting to
have my true Ingenuity to
do, whenas at Land [thro'
my continued Diligence, and
the nice Performance of my
Clock, and as without any
foolifh Obftruction or In-
terruption,]'I difcovered [or
found Means to difcover]
pretty much for the better of
late, viz. fo as whereby to
come up to fuch great Exactnefs as I fhall fpeak of below;
nor does the Watch, or will
the Watch, as by Way of
Trial, as juft here above implied, ever need any farther
than what belongs or muft

‖ And whereas, I fay, that
as touching the Thing in it
felf. no Sea Trial was at all
needful, but there did indeed.
want more Land Trials, by 2
pretty many, than what I had
had Time to make, viz. fo as
from whence to have brought
the Thing to what it is capable of bearing, but ftill it
was not fo ill as Mr Graham's
firft fetting his Pendulum a
going, and not after that, to
make any fuch Experiments,
fo as whereby to know whether or not there was any
Room-- ever to make it better, [as according to Page 14,
&c]nor could any Land Trial
of my firft Watch by a Novice,
ever direct towards making
the fame to be perfect.

belong to its adjufting, viz. as by the Help of fuch a
Clock as mine, or rather of fuch a Clock as my next
will be; and the Miftakes as here above intimated,
muft remain to other Workmen, viz. until they be as
by or from me the better inftructed, not meaning that
they fhall ever be fo inftructed, until I be [for a Public
Good] the more freely, or the more genteelly rewarded
than what I have as hitherto fneakingly been, viz for
what I had fo highly, or fo defervingly done, no, the
remaining Part of my Difcovery [and as ftill the more
valuable] fhall (excepting better Ufage) fleep, fave
only fo far as to be to my own Content or Satisfaction,
for not one Stroke as farther will I take, nor fhall I
endeavour to feek after a Place at which to prepare an
Obfervatory, with fuitable Conveniencies, for or to the
Purpofe; but as being paid fhort, and that as farther
withal,

monſtration of the Cycloid, [for that would
not ſuit the Matter at all *] it is brought
to ſuch a Degree of Perfection, as not to
gain

withal, to be attended with a great deal of Expence,
Trouble, and Hinderance, [ſcurvy Work] I will alſo
be ſhort, 'viz. as in a ſuitable Degree, excepting as intimated, I, or my Diſcoveries, can as hereafter meet
with better Uſage than what I have as heretofore met
withal , for certainly it muſt be worth all, nay more
than all the Money it was to coſt, as being ſo extraordinary a Matter, or rather, as taking in the Clock, ſuch
extraordinary Matters as were never to be expected to
have appeared in the World; no', as there is good
Reaſon to ſuppoſe, had it not been from me, would
never have ſo appeared, [as being ſo very far out of the
beaten Path] and ſtill I muſt be uſed ill, What, the
Longitude, an Affair of ſuch great Importance, and as
when to be had in ſo correct, eaſy, and uſeful a Manner, nay, as here implying more than that, and yet to
be ſo uſed ! O fie !

* That Demonſtration holding no farther good, than
as that the Spring [as they call it] at the Top of the
Pendulum, coold be ſuppoſed to be without Strength
as with reſpect to its bending or Application to the
Cycloid ; and as notwithſtanding, ſtill to be ſtrong
enough to ſuſpend the Pendulum , and that alſo, as if
the Pendulum ſhould move, or was to move by itſelf,
or of itſelf in Vacuo ; cohſequently that Demonſtration
muſt at leaſt, as with reſpect to the long Pendulum
Way, viz. where the Arch of Vibration needs not to
exceed 15 Degrees, and where, as always, or as unavoidably, the Draught of the Pendulum-Wheel of a
Clock muſt be taken into the Queſtion, muſt, I, ſay,
do more Hurt than Good, though not at all ſo to be
conſidered by Mr. Huygens, &c. yea, although in
this Point the Mathematicks or Geometry has ſo far with
Miſchief, and as only ſo to do in the Matter ; but more
of this hereafter.

gain or lofe fo much as one Second in a
Month ; * the Sufpenfion of the Pendulum
[a Thing highly material in the Matter]
being from the Brick-Wall, as having nothing to do with, or as having no Dependance from the Clock, its Cafe, or Wainfcot, for if not fo, the true Goodnefs of
what I have fhewn [or as even of more than
what I have fhewn] could not be had ; †
and

* A ftrong Proof indeed, that the Force or Draught
of the Pendulum-Wheel of my Clock, and as in the
firft Place to be underftood, with its right duly adapted Proportion, and that as partly for its Number of
Teeth, correfponding to its Revolution of 4 Minutes,
but as thence in chief, or as indifpenfably fo to be acquired thereby, [viz. from which the faid Proportion]
fuch a Qualification as whence, by my Conftruction of
the Pallats, the faid Force fo to be difpofed of, as to
give to the Pendulum no more Irregularity in the
Maintenance of its Motion in Air, than as if it went,
or could go by itfelf, fo as to be obferved to what
Truth it had continued to meafure Time, viz. as by or
from its going by itfelf, and that for a long Time in
Vacuo , and therefore I may afk, if fuch a Matter be
not highly worthy Encouragement, what other Sort of
Ingenuity or Difcovery in the World muft be fo ? my
Longitude Time-Keeper, own Sifter to this, excepted.

† For it is to be underftood, that I had, after fome
difagreeable Experiments, difcovered, that if Wood
was concerned in the Sufpenfion of the Pendulum, viz.
Wainfcot, the Clock-Cafe, [and as confequently in the
common Way, but out of the Queftion with me, the
Raifing-Board upon which the Clock ftands] the Clock
would as thence go fafter in moift Weather than in
dry, the Strength of fuch a Sufpenfion becoming as
thereby, viz by Moifture increafed, but it muft be more
or lefs fo, accordingly as the Wood may be of Strength
or

and withal (as not to pafs unnotified) the
Clock, from its Conftruction, &c. is never

to

or Subftance. Now, at fome Years after I had communicated this to Mr. Graham, he upon fome Occafion
removed a Clock from one Side of his Room to the
other, and when fixed up there, he found it to go about
6 Seconds a Day different to what it went before, and
the which, from the great Care he had taken in the Re-
moval, could be attributed from nothing fo much as
from a different Strength of the Wainfcot, but as
being very much furprifed at it, [notwithftanding what
I had communicated to him] he removed it back again
from whence he had taken it, and fixed it up there to
the fame Fixings as before, and then it went about as
what it had done before, after which [in the fame
Place] he put another Bar of Wood betwixt the Back
of the Clock-Cafe and the Wainfcot, and fcrewed the
Back faft thereto, and the Ends of the Bar (as on
Courfe) to the Wainfcot, and then it went fafter, and
the Pendulum played farther now this made or occafioned a great Alteration in Mr. Graham, viz. as
touching the whole of what he had done, for, upon
ferious Reflection, he thought that fuch as that might
not at all Times be all, but that as together from what
might pertain to the Littlenefs of his Vibration, and as
fo from the Tremor occafioned by Coaches and Carts
going by, and as with the fhutting of Doors, &c. and
as then to be in a different Place of the Room might,
as with refpect to both, have fomething to do in the
Matter, and whenas I before had certified him, that,
in a right Application of a Pendulum to a Clock, no
Alteration in its Motion could as upon any fuch Account arife, but only, as with refpect thereto, from what
the Pendulum itfelf could do, viz. as with regard to
the Strength or Stability of what it was fufpended from.
And as upon Wood, and as here by the by, the String,
or fome one Note of the String, of a Monochord, fet
exactly [as by a Leaver and Weight pertaining thereto]
to the Note or Pitch of a Bell [or, if you pleafe, of a
great Bell, as of 20 or 30 Hundred Weight] when dry
will,

to want any cleaning. * But here, as I promised above, [Page 27] it must be highly worth

will, when in moist Weather, and at the same Degree of Warmth and Tension, be sharper considerably than the said Bell, the Consequence of quicker Vibrations, viz. as then to be from a stronger Foundation, but for this Experiment, the Monochord must not be kept in a Room where there is a Fire. And here I can also as farther assert, that, as with respect to the Perfection of a single Instrument with Strings, (single, I say, because the Matter will then be the most obvious) as for Instance of that of the Viol, or at least as touching the Perfection of the same, [it being the Instrument upon which I experienced the Thing] and as in supposing its Strings to be rightly adapted to it, [or as when they are so, &c indeed] that as then for the acquiring each, or all its Notes to be to the best Perfection, that, I say, its Pitch must be set, as when in dry Weather, somewhat flatter than as when in damp, or else its Strings must be at too great a Tension in the former Case, and as I then found from Experience, its Perfection as thence to be in some Measure impaired.

* But as farther, upon due Reflection, it is certain that a Clock may still come nearer the Truth than my present Clock, the which I have here been speaking of ; and, as towards the matter, I have for some Time had such a Clock to the Purpose in great Part made ; but as not designing to fix it up in the not rightly convenient Place or House in which I live, I did not hasten its finishing , as wanting withal [viz. as lately had come in my Mind] some other or farther Experiments trying with my present going Clock, and they as to the better Completion of my other Clock, or of any such hereafter, and as when withal, Justice, as touching my Reward or Encouragement for a Public Good, was or has been the most scandalously frustrated. O fie, England ! an Act of Parliament broken, and for Sureness after twice fulfilled ; and not as only so, but that as when in the best, most compleat, or useful Manner,

VIZ.

worth notifying of how great Service the
Refiftance of the Air is, or muft be in the
Matter, viz. in its proving to give, in a
fuitably large Vibration, or in a fuitable
Largenefs of Vibration, fuch a Propernefs
of Refiftance as the Nature of the Thing
may be faid to require, for without that a
Pendulum, as under the Circumftances I
have fhewn, [viz. as with refpect to its having no fenfible Friction at the Pallats, &c.]
would know no Bounds, or at leaft but
hardly any, for its Vibrations, and confequently could never be occafioned to meafure Time truly, fince we fhall never be
able to have any Account or ufeful Obfervations about its meafuring Time, from its
going by itfelf [or as without the Wheels of
a Clock] in Vacuo; confequently it muft be
very improper for a fmall Vibration to be,
viz. where the Force from the Wheel or
Wheels

viz that is, or ever was in Nature to be wifhed for.
For, as to this Purpofe, it might have been faid as in
other Words, viz. that had fuch a Matter as in the
whole remained as Fact, it muft indeed have been a very
great Shame to the Nation , but as juft now, viz. before the publifhing of thefe Papers, the Cafe was altered ; the chief Inftruments of which Fraud, viz. the
vile holy Priefts, were over-fet, their ingenuous, or dif-
ingenuous Villainy, being at the Height, or as when
got to the Height fell, and indeed it was a very great
Fall, the Matter being got fo exceffively high , and if
they fhould rife again, yet ftill it can never be fo high
as to fee at all Times, [if ever at any Time, fo as to be
depended upon] viz. the Longitude right clear by the
Moon.

Wheels muft be but very fmall indeed, and
where as thence chiefly from a fmall Quantity of Fri&ion, and as may, for Badnefs,
be faid, *at a great Diftance from the Center
of Motion of the Pendulum*, the fame to be fo
limited, viz, for during all the Time, that
it, by the Oil, fhall chance to go, before it
[the Clock] comes to ftand, and wherein as
in Confequence thereof, [and as already im-
plied] a little Difference in the faid fmall
Fri&ion, will continually keep bearing a
great, uncertain, or irregular Proportion in
the whole Maintenance of fueh the Pendulum's feeble Motion; for though a Pendulum will, or can by proper Means, naturally
perform all its Vibrations, although of different Extent, exa&ly in equal Times, yet that
it may indeed do fo implies, that it muft not
have any the leaft Corruption from the
Wheels of a Clock, &c. and therefore, as
again, or as in Confequence of what I have
fhewn, viz. as touching the moft proper
Circumftances, no fmall Vibration can ever
to the Purpofe be rightly maintained at all;
the Refiftance of the Air, as taken into the
Queftion by a conveniently large Vibration,
[viz. convenient in other Refpe&s as well as
in this] and as when properly ballanced, or
counterballanced as above, making by far a
much better Controller or Mafter than, as
in a fmall Vibration, any little Quantity of
Fri&ion, and as with fuch Differences in
Proportion as will unavoidably happen therein,

therein, can ever with Reafon be allowed to make, or rather, as in other Words, can ever as poffibly fo be found to be; nay, if the Vibration be very fmall, it muft become even quite infipid, and not worthy of any Obfervation at all; or even when fo fmall as to be but about 2 or 3 Degrees in the whole, it could but hardly be efteemed as any better, was it not in fome Meafure to be made out by Logginefs, Maffinefs, or Exceffivenefs of Weight in the Pendulum, or even as it were in other Words, by an enormous Weight in the Bob; but indeed, as fo, it may or might [as with a Provifion for Heat and Cold, or as with fomething greatly towards the Effects thereof] do better by much than what had been done before, but ftill certainly, it cannot be taken as a Wonder, if a little Difference in Glibnefs or Clamminefs upon the Surface of fuch Pallats, and as at fuch a great Diftance from the Center of Motion of the Pendulum, viz. as Mr. Graham difpofed it, and as together with fuch his coincident feeble Vibration, I fay, it cannot be taken as a Wonder, but that the Clock may vary, as thence by Times a Second in a Day, whenas, if proper Steps be taken, *or can be taken,* in or for the adjufting my next Clock, there muft be then more Reafon (and that withal, as from Experience in my other Clock) that it fhall perform to a Second in 100 Days, yea, I fay, more Reafon, than

that

that Mr. Graham's fhould perform to a Second in 1. And now how far, or to what Equality, the Properties treated of above, viz. as touching my Pendulum-Clock, are preferved in my Watch, or, Time-Keeper for the Longitude, may in fome Meafure be obferved as followeth.

As firft, 'the Radius of its Ballance, as with refpeƈt to that of the Circle, the Portion of which the Edge of its Pallats defcribe, is about as 32 to 1, * fo it is in Effeƈt, from Propernefs of Weight in the Rim of the faid Ballance, and Strength of the Ballance-Spring, [the Strength of which Spring as below, producing more Force than what natural Gravity as in a Pendulum can do] and as together with the Largenefs of the Arch which the Ballance fetches or defcribes, viz. as about 255 Degrees, and that 5 Times in a Second, and as withal from the fmall Force it has from, or its little Concernment with the Wheel, [not meaning very little or fmall in itfelf, or inconfiftently fmall, as liking in Faƈt to a Creature that's fick and unaƈtive, or as according to Mr. Graham's Way for the Pendulum, but only as properly, or as it were reciprocally fmall, in regard to the Smallnefs of the Diftance at which the Wheel acts from the Center of
the

* The Radius of the Ballance being 1 ⅛ Inch, *i. e.* in a Deccmal 1.125 Inch, and that of the Pallats 0.035 Inch

the Ballance, viz. as with refpect to the
Radius of the fame, its Weight and Arch, or
rather Arches defcribing] there muft, I fay,
be in Effect, a much longer Pendulum, or
fuch a Thing as muft have a much greater
Power whereby to regulate, than Mr.
Graham's Pendulum that fwings, or rather
creeps, as he managed the Matter Seconds;
natural Gravity exerting but very little
Force there, [viz. as towards the Matter of
Truth in Mr. Graham's Pendulum] as being improperly, more to be compared to the
Motion of a Comet in its Aphelion, [i. e. fo
as that a little may difturb or alter it] than
to the Motion of a Planet in any Part of its
Orbit, and as whence to be looked upon, as
feemingly a Matter fo contrived, as if it was
for fear the Pendulum fhould do any Good,
yea, rather than it fhould do any, viz. as
when confidered in a right Light or Manner;
for, as otherwife to the fame Signification,
the lefs the Vibration of any Pendulum, viz.
whether heavy or light, the more in Nature
it muft debafe, approach or decline towards
the bad Effect of a Ballance of fuch the
fame Weight, &c. and as with fuch the
fame infignificantly fmall Vibration; and
indeed as fo, and as together with what
bid I have fhewn as farther, or as ftill naturally to attend it, was I to fet up fuch a
Clock, and in the Manner in which they
commonly are fet up, I could but, as from
the Nature of the Thing fay, that I had only

fet

set it up, in order [as for a rude Trial] to see
how it should chance (as according to Lord
Morton) to go, or to continue in its Mensuration of Time, viz. as with regard to the
Matter of Exactness.

Now in my Longitude Time-Keeper,
[pursuant to what has been said] the Strength
or Command which the Ballance-Spring
has over the Ballance, as in Proportion to
the Force it has from the Wheel, is so great
as 80, or even as more than 80 to 1; a
strong artificial Gravity indeed, [for so it
may be termed] as even in Effect---much
surpassing natural; * whenas, as barely in
which Respect, viz. besides the other ne-
cessary or very material Circumstances at-
tending, or the which ought to attend, [as
correspondent to what I have said of my
Pallats

---

* The Limb of the Ballance moving thereby through
about 25 Inches in a Second, notwithstanding, as in
that Time [and as still an Augmentation to its Power
or Dominion] its Motion being changed to contrary
Direction 5 Times, and as from which it must as in
Consequence be as farther allowed, and as withal consi-
dering the Arch it describes, that its Motion must be
prodigiously quick, or even violently powerful in the
Middle of each Vibration, and when, as even without
that, 25 Inches in a Second, is no less than 34 Miles
a Day, so rapid and powerful is the Motion of the
Ballance, for faint sleepy Work could never do, and
whenas no such Velocity [as in this Point for the bet-
ter] can be in a Pendulum, viz. in such Arches as in
the long Pendulum Way are commonly, or can as the
most properly be described, until it comes to about the
Length of 13 Foot, and then it will still not be in Effect

Pallats' for the Pendulum, and of which
there was no Notion in the World before,
but of the Manner of which as touching
the Watch, neither of that of my Provifion
therein for Heat and Cold, I fhall not here
treat or enlarge] they never did in the common Way, nor, as there is good Reafon to
fuppofe,

fect fo quick, nor confequently fo powerful, becaufe of
its not having as in Effect fo much Velocity, but only
fo much as whereby to accomplifh a Vibration, or fuch
a Space, viz. as without any Returns or Return, in
the Space of two Seconds of
Time; ‖ but here, if it fhould

|| But ftill, as by the by, it
may be noted, that there can
be no Occafion for a Pendulum for any Church Clock
whatever, to be any longer
than as to fwing 2 Seconds.

be alledged, that the Length
of fuch a Pendulum is much
longer than the Radius of
this Ballance, it is then to be
remembered, that (as in common) the Lengths of the
Pallats, &c. are to be taken into the Queftion , and, as
already in fome Meafure implied, it is as farther to be
underftood or remembered, that in fuch---thefe mechanical Cafes, that no Ponderofity in a Pendulum or a
Ballance, can rightly or ever make up---the Want of
Velocity , and indeed Velocity was very much wanting
in my three large Machines, yea, I fay, very much,
notwithftanding their Weightinefs of Ballances, or as
notwithftanding what Philofophers may reafon in other
Affairs, or rather what Philofophy in this Affair [viz.
as hitherto through Miftake, as from the Steel-Yard,
&c. in the Matter] might teach us to reafon , but I
did not then [viz. as in the Defigns of my three large
Machines] fo thoroughly underftand it, nor fhould I,
or the World, (as I think I may make bold to fay) ever
have underftood it, had it not been, or had I not difcovered it as it were through Accident, in or by my
third Machine , but as it would be, more tedious here
than neceffary, for me to fully reafon the Matter, I fhall
forbear it, but ftill the Knowledge of the fame is highly
material.

fuppofe, ever would have exceeded in this grand Point, [viz in the Quantity of Force which the Ballance has from its Spring, as in Proportion to what it has from' the Wheel] any more than as about 3 to 1; not that any, either amongft the Watch-Makers, or Men of liberal Sciences, were able, or had in the leaft confidered, how far indeed, as towards fuch a Matter, they only had, or there only was advanced; confequently, as touching the Point, had never found any Occafion to confider, whether or not they might ever be able by any Means poffible, to advance any higher, [viz before that fome of them had heard me fpeak about it] or rather, whether or not it was, or could be at all material, for it fo to be, viz. in this ---the moft material Circumftance, any higher or farther advanced, and that in fuch a Bulk or Size of a Watch, as might for the Purpofe be the moft conveniently chofen; whenas, without which, no Provifion for Heat and Cold, &c. [had any fuch Thing withal been thought to have been wanting] could ever be, or could ever have been, of any true Service in the Affair. But here it may not be amifs for me to remark, that after I had difcovered, viz. by doing fomething as by Way of Trial towards this Matter, that it was after a many toilfome Experiments or Alterations, that I did indeed fucceed to fuch a furprifing Degree as I did, a ftrange Difference for the better, being

betwixt

betwixt 80 to 1, and 3 to 1 ! I fay, this was attained by a great deal of Labour, but it was fo as wherein withal [and as with a great Vibration] to be thoroughly fatisfied, that it was, or is, as far as poffible---to be acquired or done; fo therefore, if Mr. Mafkelyne fhould [after a long Time] find an Equivalent, it is not poffible for him to go any farther.

And now that this great or chief Matter as above, is indeed fo much as 80 to 1, is to be underftood or perceived as followeth, viz. as in that from the Force of the Ballance-Wheel alone, *i. e.* as without the Ballance-Spring, the Ballance will be almoft 2 Seconds in fetching 1 Vibration, whenas, with its Spring, it fetches 10 Vibrations in 2 Seconds, and it is certain that different Velocities are, or muft be, as the fquare Roots of their Forces; confequently if the Ballance, without its Spring, or without as it were its artificial Gravity, took up 2 Seconds, wherein to fetch 1 Vibration, and wherein it fetches 10, the Wheel would then but have the $\frac{1}{100}$ Part of its Command; but here it is as farther withal to be notified, that if, or as when at any Time, any fmall Difference happens therein, viz. in the faid eightieth Part, as indeed fmall, or even as almoft infinitely fmall, fuch a Matter muft be, or can but be, as with refpect to the whole Force of the Ballance, yet ftill, I fay, the fame as in the fame Contrivance, to be taken

taken in or accounted for ; hence, as ftill
farther concerning this Matter, or rather
now, as unconcerning the fame, and that befides what might have ever arofe from the
common Experiments of Workmen, viz.
nothing, there is not, nor could ever have
been at y likelihood, as above intimated,
that any Affiftance or Difcovery herein
fhould ever have fhewn itfelf, or appeared to
the World from fuch mechanical Illuftrations
or Operations as they exhibit at Cambridge,
Oxford, &c. as being indeed for the moft
Part only fuch Experiments as need not at
all to be tried, [Hornbook Work as it were]
but as granting them ufeful in the moft
common Refpects, they could never however have had any Thing to do with this
Difcovery of mine, as being as it were quite
repugnant to them, or at leaft quite out of
the Run of that Channel ; but ftill, or as
notwithftanding, as fuch weak, or even very
weak Mechanicks as touching this Matter,
viz. fuch as neither know, nor can be made
to know any Thing of the Matter, * but
yet muft, as in the moft ftupendous, but fur-
feiting

---

* For in particular, I took fome Pains with Mr.
Shepherd, [viz. when he was my Friend] but could
make nothing of him, [viz. any farther than that one
Wheel turned another] although it was at his Defire.
Very unfit Gentlemen to be my Mafters, the Reward
for the Longitude [I mean Part thereof] being to be
detained in their fecret Clofets for during their Pleafure,
as having in, or for that Interim, a pretty Reward ;
but

feiting Manner, be my Maſters ! But then
as ſo, it may as in Conſequence be ſaid or
aſked, what was there to be expected ? and
as when moreover, as at the ſame Time, or
all the while to be Rivals and Antag... is,
by another Way as they would have it for
the Longitude, viz. as by the ſlow and in-
tricate Motion of the Moon, and as whence,
or wherein to be attended with great Difficulties and Uncertainties in the making Obſervations, and conſequently the Reſult to
be for the moſt Part attended with very great
Error, inſomuch, (and as without the taking
any Notice of ſuch—the operoſe Calculations that muſt be required) that from the
Experience which Dr. Halley had had in
the Matter, it ſo, or at laſt appeared, or
was found by him, that if in Caſe the Lunar
Tables were ever ſo correct, that even ſtill,
as from the Obſervations alone, [viz. when
they could be had] there could no certain
Good ever come from that Way to work,
viz. ſo as to be relied on, and upon which
Account

but as notwithſtanding they took great Care about my
Watch, for they alſo locked it up for ſome Months in a
Cloſet at the Admiralty,—becauſe it had performed two
Voyages ſo well , and ſo they would keep it as a Piece
of Treaſure, for fear nobody elſe ſhould ever be able to
make ſuch another , a fair Sign indeed, that they did
not underſtand it, and conſequently to be taken as an
Abſurdity that they ſhould (at that Rate) have had
any Thing to do with it , but, to make it worſe, Lord
Morton, for want of underſtanding as well as they,
put or infuſed Chance into their Heads. *see an ad-*
dition p. 109.

Account chiefly it was, as Mr. Graham told me, that he [viz. Dr. Halley] ceafed his Purfuit in the Matter, an ingenuous Decifion indeed, [fince, as already implied, no Proceeding therein or thereby could ever with any Certainty tend to a Public Good] for it is ftill certain, that fuch Obfervations cannot be any better made now, neither with any more Frequency be had, than could be then, viz. in Dr. Halley's Time.

Now, from Experience, I can make bold to fay, that my Watch [or Time-Keeper for the Longitude] will come up to 1 Second in a Fortnight, viz. as when my laft Piece of Improvement, and as with a little Alteration, viz. fo as whereby to receive it, is put in Execution, * the which I defcribed in Drawings in the latter End of the Year of our Lord 1772, and as then in the 80th Year of my Age; and furely it ought to be looked upon as an Age well fpent, † as tending

---

* The which Improvement being to be in the Parts which are above (as Work-men termed it) the Upper-Plate of the Watch, and as with a little Alteration in the Shape of the Pallats, but as eafier for the future, in all Refpects to be done, as well as when done to afford a greater Degree of Truth.

† Confidering what tedious Proceedings, in or for Experiments, belonging to this muft be required, viz. fo as to purchafe, or to find out the fecret Way, [or rather fome Secrets in the Way, and them as the only true Steps] fo as whereby to make a thorough Conqueft of the Thing; nothing to the Matter being done before!

tending fo highly to a Public Good, [*i. e.* if it may be fo let to do] as well as to the making hereafter a pretty Employment for ingenious Men, though not for Priefts at Cambridge and Oxford.

Now I promifed above to fay fomething farther as with refpect to the Pendulum. I have faid that Mr. Huygens's Demon-ftration of the Cycloid can be of no Service in the Affair, viz. no farther than as if it was to be fuppofed in Vacuo, &c. if that may be faid to be of Service ; and when as [whether in Vacuo or not] was it to be applied [ac-cordingly as demonftrated] to a very thin Spring at the Top of the Pendulum, [for thin to the Purpofe it muft be] * it would only occafion the faid Spring to neck, or break off at the Top of the Cycloid, and that in a fhort Time ; nor can the Arch or Arches, as defcribed in the long Pendulum Way, [as fuppofing at the moft 15 Degrees] be but hardly faid to want it, [viz. as in the Manner demonftrated] therefore fuch a Matter as muft be in lieu of what is called a Cycloid, muft be chiefly to preferve the Spring [or Sufpenfion of the Pendulum] from its ever breaking, and the which Spring, as being to be very thin, (but may be

---

* Confequently the Pendulum here not to be fo monftroufly heavy as according to Mr. Graham, the Thinnefs of the Spring not to bear with that, neither does Nature befpeak it fo to be, but that, as on the other Hand, or as in the moft natural Courfe otherwife.

be ſhort) muſt be beſt to be made of Gold, *
properly allayed with Copper, and to be
well hammered before it be brought to its
Thinneſs, [as being then more elaſtic, than
as if or when allayed with Silver] Now
the Nature of ſuch a Matter, or Cycloid to
the Purpoſe, [and as conſequently withal
for preſerving the Spring] muſt be as in
ſome Meaſure reverſe to what is demon-
ſtrated by Mr. Huygens, &c. that is, it muſt
be ſo as to occaſion little Vibrations of the
Pendulum, viz all ſuch as are leſs (and
unregarded) than ſo as to let, or ſuch as will
let the Pallats interchange, to be ſtill ſooner
performed, than what they would as otherwiſe be without it; and at ſuch an Arch
deſcribing, as whereby juſt to let the Pallats
interchange, or as rather at a little bigger,
the Length of the Pendulum to be ſo [viz.
as by or from its adjuſting] as then to ſwing
Seconds, and alſo, as when in its fetching
farther [as from the Nature of ſuch a Cycloid as muſt be, and as when together upon
ſuch other Foundation as above deſcribed]
the ſame; for as thence, from the Continuation of the circular Curvature of the
Cheeks, [viz. of this artificial Cycloid] that
Matter, as here in Hand, is to be aſcertained, but of the Radius, in each to the
Purpoſe,

---

* And withal (as here by the by) the Pin, on which
the Pallats [as of Wood] have their relative Motion,
and that as with Friction inſenſible to the Pendulum,
as I have ſhewn.

Purpofe, viz. as fubfequent to the Action of
the Pallats I fhall not here fpeak, nor can
Cambridge and Oxford Education have any
Thing to do with either that or the Action
of the faid Pallats, [viz. fo as to define fuch
a Matter or Matters to Exactnefs, had fuch
Particulars as them ever before been thought
of; but however, as each Check, with regard to the Property I have fhewn of the
Pallats, or as a Tenor to their Refult, muft
be the Arch of a Circle, [viz. for fo far as
will, in this material Point, be fuitably
wanted or ufed, *i. e.* befides an Overplus of
the fame for its more truly making] it can
be done to a mathematical Truth, whenas
the other (as according to Mr. Huygens)
could not, was it fo to be wanted. So now
to the Purpofe it is to be underftood, that
from the Force or Draught of the Pendulum-Wheel, as being by the Pallats properly difpofed of, [viz. as according to the
Note, Page 25] and as wherein with a proper recoiling of the fame, that the Cycloid
may be fo, as that when the faid Wheel
may have [or as when in occafioning the faid
Wheel to have] fomewhat a greater Force,
I fay the Vibrations of the Pendulum, as
thence becoming bigger, may ftill be performed exactly in the fame Time, and as
alfo the fame when the Air gives or may
give fomewhat a leffer Refiftance to the
Pendulum, fo that its Vibrations become
fomewhat greater without any more Force
from

from the Wheel, and this, becaufe for the moft part, that from the fame Caufe which will leffen the Refiftance of the Air, the Pendulum is to become in itfelf, as mathematically fpeaking, fhorter; and indeed, from the whole of what I have fhewn, a great Exactnefs in the meafuring of Time is to be had ; for withal, it is to be confidered, that the Draught or Force of the Pendulum-Wheel, in my Sort of Clock-Work, will alter but very little, neither the Vibration of the Pendulum, as from thence, or any other Caufe, much at any Time, or in any Sort of Weather; fo no Wonder certainly [as from the whole] at the nice Performance of fuch a Clock, or fine Contrivance of Mechanifm, as the which was indeed to the Aftonifhment of my great and worthy Friend Mr. Graham ; and it is certain, that the Refult of fuch as this [viz. as when to be had from a Watch—rightly or thoroughly converted] muft be the neareft Relation to the Longitude, nay, even from its eafy and proper Application—the Longitude ; and yet they that muft be my Mafters, know nothing at all of the Matter, [viz. of fuch Mechanifm] * it being as

it

---

* But as notwithftanding will ftill, as by Pretence of Trial, and through the Power invefted in them, employ any who know as little of it, or about fuch Mechanifm as they themfelves do, an evil Cafe fure ! Their Cambridge and Oxford Mechanicks (as above) not reaching that, [the very Soul as it were of the Matter]

it were not only repugnant to their Learning, but withal, as they imagine, the Lofs
of a Booty to them, for Dr. Bradley once
faid to me, that if it had not been for my
Watch, * that he, as jointly with Mr. Ir-
winn, (and, I may fay, as Opportunity of Ignorance then ferved) could have had 10000l.
and fo my Mafters [or rather improper In-
fpectors]

ter] but as on the other Hand, or rather as on the contrary, have writ and publifhed a great deal of Stuff,
pertaining, as they think, to the Longitude, or at leaft
would have others fo to believe it to be, whenas it is
ftill no farther than as what Mr Whifton did, viz. by
his throwing up a Bomb [in the dark] at Shooter's-Hill,
[as taking Occafion fo to do foon after I came] for the
which only made or could make a great Noife, and the
Greatnefs or Impertinence or their Superfluity, as not
having any Thing to do in the Matter, [viz. as in their
Nautical Almanac] can do no better ; for, as touching
the fame, was they to be afked, what is the ufeful Intent
at Sea of fuch a Column therein, or fuch a Column, or
fuch a Column, nay even to 40, &c. in a Month or
each Month, their Anfwer in the main could be no
better than nothing ! as being only a deal of Stuff, fo
as whereby to dazzle the World, for though ever fo
true in itfelf, can have nothing to do with the Longitude at Sea ! O ftrange, that any of the Commiffioners
fhould fuffer themfelves to be fo impofed upon ! I wifh
not only they, but that all the Nation underftood it as
well as I do.

   * The which, by the by, I believe was his Death,
becaufe he, as the only one amongft them, did indeed,
from his oft converfing with me, and Sagacity in the
Matter, underftand it, viz. what it was likely to do,
but ftill (as previous to his Conjunction with Mr. Ir-
winn) feemed to be very forry when I met with any
Difficulty, as chiefly in that of the Diamond Pallats.
No Difficulty now.

fpe{tor$] would ftill have People to be in
Love with fuch other Things as wherein to
make the beft of [viz. as without the taking
any Notice of the great Trouble attending]
muft, at leaft, be far more, if not even a
Hundred Times more difficult to tell to a
Degree of Longitude, and that only when
Opportnnities may happen, and fuch as will
but be feldom, than to tell what's o'Clock
to a Minute by the Hour-Hand of a Watch.
This cannot be denied by any. But as here
to return to the Clock, it muft be indeed, as
at firft to get fuch a Clock to be really or
truly adjufted, *i. e.* to what it will bear, or
is capable of bearing, viz. as without another of the fame Sort---no eafy Matter to
be done * and that becaufe of Deficiency in,

as

* There being to be concerned in that Proceeding,
four different Things, and wherein two of which (as
touching the Point) do as it were pretty much confpire
to, or in the fame Purpofe, viz. the Compofers of the
Pallets to relative Reft, and the correfpondent Curvature thereto of the Cycloid Cheeks. I fay, thefe two
Things may only as almoft be taken as one, viz. in
their joint Effects, for fo far as belongs to this Matter,
but not quite fo, and the other two Particulars in the
Cafe, are the adjufting [viz. by a proper Provifion]
the Wires, or the redoubling of the Wires for Heat and
Cold in the Pendulum, and the Screw for faft and flow
in general at the Bottom of the Pendulum. And as
hence I may fay, as Rectifications in thefe different
Things muft pertain to the Clock's adjufting, (viz as
at firft by the Mafter Workman) it is or muft as therefore be a Thing—quite impoffible to be done to Exactnefs or Perfection, by or from any celeftial Obfervations
whatever,

as well as Scarcity of Celeſtial Obſervations,
as not being in the Time of adjuſting, neither with Frequency nor Exactneſs to be
had, viz. as when moſt to the Purpoſe
wanting. Now this is meaning, as without
what is to be done by the Screw at the
Bottom of the Pendulum, viz. for faſt and
ſlow in general, that being an eaſy Matter,
viz. when the others are really done ; but
when, as after once in that, as well as to be
in the firſt Place, in other Reſpects adjuſted,
and to ſtand in the ſame, but proper Place,
it will 'hold to its Truth, as I ſuppoſe, or
have, from Experience, Reaſon to believe)
for Ages ; * not meaning but that it may |
be removed from the Place, or a Place of |
Convenience, wherein as at firſt to be ad-
·juſted, viz. by the Maker, &c. to any other
proper Place, and there or then [viz. after
duly fixed up, or as in other Words, after a
firm and ſkilful fixing] to be as again ad-
E juſted,

whatever, no, nor indeed by or from any other Means
whatever, unleſs [as here meaning of Courſe] the Foundation and principal Parts, or rather Principles of the
Clock be to the Purpoſe as I have ſhewn, and could as
thence ſtill farther ſhew.

* But here, as by the by, I may notify, that a Pro-
feſſor, as great as any of the reſt, and who rudely made
an Application to me for a
‖ Viz. one of my Maſters Clock, ‖ muſt little think, as
at the Board of Longitude. from their Shortneſs in the
Matter, and great Abuſe of
me of what really ought to belong to the having an
Aſtronomical Clock, or as otherwiſe to that Purpoſ
nothing,

justed, viz. as with respect to fast and slow in general, as the Latitude of the Place may require; and the which (as above) no great Difficulty; whenas the first, as the far more essential Part or Parts of adjusting, must be very difficult, viz. as when alone to be done without another such Clock, and that as the best when already adjusted, and so as whereby, by the seeing of both the Pendulums as it were instant, and as when at the same Time, the Clocks to be the most properly placed, viz. one in one Room, and the other in another, * yet still, as intimated, to be

at

nothing; for [as otherwise with Respect to the same] I am very sure, that I should then neither think it, nor find it worth any thing at all in the Affair. ‖ But how the Nation [or World] must, or will fairly come at what is much better, or truly fit for this Purpose, ought to be fairly or rightly considered,

‖ They can indeed tell us of what will be the Result of the Motion or Motions of two Marbles [such as Boys play withal] rapping or impinging one against the other.

not but that I once thought of giving a Clock to the Observatory at Greenwich, but my bad Usage proved too tedious for that , but still, as already hinted, my next or second Clock will be somewhat better than if it had been finished sooner , and if I live to see it done, that will be my Wages in the Matter; but one would think, a Minstrel at the Play-House is much better off, save only that this has been my great Delight, and must be more noble than his Atchievements.

* A Chimney being in each, so that either one of which Rooms may be made warm with Fire, viz. when properly so to be wanted , and then, if indeed neither of the Clocks was adjusted, it would be no great Difficulty to get them both so.

at any Time, viz. as by a little turning of
the Eyes in the Door-stead, (the Door of
each Clock-case being opened for the Purpose) compared to the 20th Part of a Second,
or less; but as when (and as very troublesome and tedious) without this, a right Re-
course to the Stars, the right Ascension of
such, as may be the most proper, here to
observe by, being to be as yearly known,
or even if not known, yet, as the Rate of
the Clock's going may as thence be ascer-
tained, viz. as nearly as such deficient Observations [viz. as with respect to this Pur-
pose] can be taken or had, must be better
than the Sun; whence it is still highly to be
remembered, that this can never be so easily,
nor so well accomplished, as when by or
from the two Clocks; no, such Observations can only serve or suit for the trying
and correcting such Clocks as Mr. Graham's,
but as whence to adjust a Clock to Perfection, [i. e. meaning such a Clock as will
bear in good Earnest so to be done by]
could never as thence be done in an Age;
the Stars indeed will do better than the Sun,
the Equation Tables not being as yet right,
no, not in our late famous, or rather [as to
its Design] infamous Nautical Almanac,
neither, as already implied, can any celestial
Observation ever be so correctly or so strictly
made, as not only, for this Matter ought to
be, but that as withal, when most to the
Purpose wanted; whenas, by a right Use of

my

my Clocks, [viz. as when with proper Con-
veniences, and proper Apparatuffes] even
that Piece of Aftronomy [the Equation]
may hereafter be corrected, becaufe as thence
the Eccentricity of the Earth's Orbit, and
whatever elfe may pertain to the Matter,
may be the better known. But it is to be
underftood, that my Watch in its Perfection
[and as without any Trouble of fixing, and
not as obli fo, but as partly withal, as
thence to be attended with far more, or farther Ufefulnefs, in different Places than the
Clock] would be the beft for a Tranfit of
Venus, &c was there, or be there fuch a
Matter as ftill or as again to be thought to
be wanted.

And now, if the Royal Society pleafe, I
will fhew them the Draught of the Clock
which I have in great Part made, and not
only the Draught of the Pallats, as in particular, but alfo the Pallats themfelves, in
order that they may fee at leaft fome Reafon for what I found, or might as in Confequence find from fuch a Contrivance of
Pallats; but not meaning as only from the
extraordinary Qualification of, or in the
fame, but as together from other Things,
and as befides them the which I have treated
of; but ftill, I fay, the indifpenfable Conftruction of the faid Pallats, viz. for their
Duty as above, and as muft in Confequence,
or good Reafon, be with or from due Propernefs in the Extenfion of the Periphery of

the

the Pendulum-Wheel, and the Number of
Teeth in the fame, [viz. as then anfwerable,
in its beating Seconds, to its Revolution of
4 Minutes] for otherwife (as prefuppofed in
the Note, beginning on Page 25) they could
not do their Duty, viz. in their fo properly
acting upon the Pendulum, as muft for a nice,
or true Performance, or as in other Words,
for a conftantly ftrict Menfuration of Time .
be required; * whence they the faid Pallats
muft, I fay, amongft the reft, be to the Purpofe by far the moft principal; and this my
great and worthy Friend Mr. Folkes, in his
Speech to the Royal Society, [30th Novem-
ber, 1749] in fome Meafure reprefented;
but certainly it muft, from what I have
fhewn, be fairly vifible, that as in Comparifon thereof, and withal as taking in the bad
Circumftance of Oil, or Difference in Friction [was it, or could it be even without
Oil] at fuch a great Diftance from the Center

* And wherein as withal to be obferved, (as intimated Page 11) that the Wheel is but to move a little in
a Second, [as half the Space of one of its Teeth, the
which are but ftraight] but the Pendulum through a
great Space. But here, as without taking any Notice
of this material Matter the Vibration, it is to be remembered, that the Length of a Pendulum, as at the
heft, is only as in Proportion to the Length of the
Pallats, or as more properly to the Diftance at which
the Wheel acts from the Center of Motion of the Pendulum, viz. as without any Thing to be taken as farther therein for the worfe, as the which is ftill fo to be
notified in Mr. Graham's Cafe, and that as not in
a fmall Degree.

ter of Motion of the Pendulum, as in Mr. Graham's Way, and as together with the Smallnefs of the Vibration as cohering therewith, that it cannot (I fay) be otherwife looked upon, but as a Matter or Matters quite ridiculous, as being even quite repugnant to Reafon ; but a Pendulum, with a Provifion for Heat and Cold, and from a firm Sufpenfion, muft do fomething, but certainly in or towards which natural Property, it cannot be faid that Mr. Graham's Pallats can do any Thing, for no worfe Thing could well be contrived than they are, as being only as it were a meer jerting, ftamping, nonfenfical Fancy, * as if fo defigned, as that the Clock might as thence the better be heard to go, as if no Matter how it went, or was to go ; I fay this muft feemingly be the Cafe, whatever Occafion he might take as otherwife at firft to think about them ; and in the whole, as in Comparifon to the Account I have given of mine, one

* And yet the fame to have taken fuch thorough Root or Poffeffion in Men's Minds, as that, whatever any Man may contrive or do, it muft be a-kin thereto, or otherwife, the firft Obfervation or Cry will be, that it does not beat dead ! a furprifing Circumftance indeed ! as having nothing at all to do in the Matter, viz. as with refpect to what muft be done, fo as to afford the Truth, and confequently fo as not to corrupt, or as in the leaft to baffle, the natural Qualifications of the Pendulum, but as that it may have all its advantageous Properties to the Purpofe, as from Largenefs of Vibration, &c. as I have fhewn.

one would think the fame muft be vifibly
bad to any of Judgment, and as even without Experience, [no ftrict Regularity, as I
have 'fhewn, being as thence with Reafon
to be expected or afforded, at' leaft for any
Continuation of Time.] But now, as farther, (and as according to my fame worthy
Friend Mr. Folkes's Prediction) it certainly
is as ftill more highly to be notified, viz.
the Conftruction of the Pallats of my now
fmall Machine, Watch, or Time-Keeper
for the Longitude, * and efpecially as in my
laft Drawing, viz. fo as wherein or whereby
exactly to fuit in each or all Refpects, as well
as my other Pallats, to the Nature or Property of a Pendulum, [viz. more properly
than as in my firft Watch, nay, fomewhat
better, or more to the Purpofe, than as at
prefent in my fecond Watch] and ftill as
not to pafs unnotified, the Materials of
which the Ballance-Wheel and Pallats refpectively are made, viz. the Wheel of Steel,
quite hard, and the Pallats of Diamond, and
as whence, fo far as I am hitherto able to
judge, they will hold to their Figures for
Ages; neither will the Watch in any other
Refpect [but as chiefly from my laft Drawing,

---

* Viz where the Vibration, or as Workmen, term it
Croffing, muft to the Purpofe be very large, and fo as
thence confequently, from its 5 Vibrations in a Second,
the Weight, but as more efpecially from the Largenefs
of the Diameter of the Ballance, its Motion to be very
quick and powerful, or even as it were boifterous, as I
have fhewn above, Page 38.

ing, and where the Pallats will also be somewhat easier to be done] hardly ever be out
of Order, but as above, to point out the
Time [and that whether at Sea or Land] to a
Second in a Fortnight; and had not my
Proceedings been foolishly baffled, this our
Nation might certainly have had some Be-
nefit from them before this Time; but as
on the contrary, meeting with such extremely ill Treatment, I did, for some Time,---
even hate to think of so much as ever any
more to occasion one Wheel to turn another, whenas there is a great deal more than
what that contains to, to be thought about
in the Matter; but, alas! it is to be sup-
posed, as a great Advantage for such ill
Treatment [or bad Matter] to be, was my
being neither University-man, Knight nor
Earl, &c. insomuch, that even an Act of
Parliament could not possibly, or at least,
not so well, as on my Behalf stand good;
but still I had not, nor must not have any
Intelligence whether it would or not---until
some Time after my Son was returned from
his second Voyage, notwithstanding his being sent upon both his Voyages by Virtue
of the said Act, and the Longitude [by my
Time-Keeper] to be had in each or both of
them, even to much nearer the Truth than
what by the same was required! A fine
Commendation sure to the Nation, viz. in
one Respect, but quite the contrary in another. But had it been possible that the
Professors

Profeffors of Arts or Sciences at Cambridge
and Oxford, as from their high Algebra,
&c.* could have been able to have difcovered
or to have comprehended fuch Mechanifm
to have been in Nature, as I am now, by
the Bleffing of God, Mafter of, viz. for
Time-keeping, and I to have been apprifed
of it, [viz. of their knowing that] and ftill,
or as notwithftanding, to have come out of
the Country from where I did come, and as
with a Scheme or Defcription for finding
the Longitude by the Moon, and as when
the Ufe of which muft, and as even at the
beft, or feldom Opportunities ftand, or rather turn upon fuch tickle Points or Uncertainties as it muft do, † and of which the
Profeffors muft hardly, or prefumptuoufly
be faid to be ignorant ; what a Fool of a
Fellow muft I then have been ! yea even fo,
as neither to have been heard to fpeak to
Mr. Graham, nor to any body elfe, viz. of
any underftanding in the Matter , but however, be it now as it will, if it fo pleafe Almighty God, to continue my Life and
Health

---

* Not from Divinity, by which they wear their
Gowns, for that would but hardly have let them to
have, or ever to have had any Thing to do in the Matter.

† And for which Reafon as above, [Page 44] Dr.
Halley gave it over , and as being pleafed that fuch a
Thing as mine was [to a Public Good] likely to do, [or
to be brought to bear] promifed to Mr. Graham, that,
as in Confequence thereof, he would attend the Board
of Longitude, rain, fnow, or blow,

Health a little longer, they the Profeffors
[or Priefts] fhall not hinder me of my Pleafure, as from my laft Drawing, viz. of
bringing my Watch to a Second in a Fortnight, I fay I am refolved of this, though
quite unfuitable to the Ufage I have had, or
was ever to expect from them ; and whenas Dr. Bradley once faid to me, [not but
that I underftood the fame without his faying it] viz. that if Time-keeping could be
to 10 Seconds in a Week, it would, as with
refpect to the Longitude, be much prefer-
able to any other way or Method. And
fo, as I do not now mind the Money, [as
not having Occafion fo to do, and withal as
being weary of that] the Devil may take
the Priefts ; for Dr. Bradley owned to me,
that as otherwife in the Matter, there might
be always Error in the Tables ; always Error, viz. in fome Refpect or other in the
making or preparing an Inftrument; always Error in the obferving; and always
Error from the Refraction ; and as moreover owned, that as full in the whole, a little Variation from the Truth [and as without taking any Notice of what was to come
from the Performance of a common Watch,
its fetting, &c.] might be of extremely ill
Confequence in the Affair ; and yet it
feemed that, for the Love of Money, he
could even have broke through all ! And
now the Parfons ftill want to prefer fuch the
fame Method for the Longitude, viz. fuch

as

as will always be attended with very great
Difficulties and Uncertainties, and besides
the very troublesome and tedious Calculations, which must as thereunto belong, and
as wherein to be liable to Mistake, * and
consequently may sometimes or often times,
as from the whole, be attended with great
Damage; I say, for the Love of Money,
they the Professors or Priests want to prefer
this, above what may be done with Ease
and Pleasure, and with pretty great Frequency to a great Degree of Exactness, [for
if the Love of Money cannot be said to be
the Case, they must be no better than as if
out of their Senses, for certainly Parsons
would never concern themselves at such a
Rate, or in such a Manner, if Money was
not at the Bottom.] But now, as Experience in any Thing is the best Proof of its
Usefulness, Goodness, &c.---When Mr.
Charles Green [one of the best Observers]
and my Son came together from Barbadoes,
along with Captain Manley, and though for
the most Part fine Weather during the
Voyage, yet Mr. Green, as only on the Day
Time, attempted to make Observations, and
that as at the Time, or at such a Time as
when the Sun and Moon were in such Situ-
ation with Respect to each other, viz. as
when

---

* As was the Case in one of the two Observations,
the which Mr. Green could only make as below, [as
was proved so to be from my Watch] and through
which Mistake, he sweat at his Figures for some Hours.

when in Diſtance betwixt 40 Degrees and
100, or not much exceeding either Way,
and as when, in the ſaid Time, the Horizon
happened to be, or to prove, right properly
clear for the Purpoſe, and as then, from his
making ſeveral Attempts, viz. as only in that
advantageous Caſe, or ſeldom Opportunity,
(no Attempt by the Stars to be made, although as the moſt from thence to be
wanted, for if there had, or he had made
any ſuch Attempt, it would have been much
worſe, my Watch being there) got in all
with much Difficulty, two Obſervations,
whenas, in the whole Voyage, there were
but 3 or 4 Days on which my Son could not
as with Eaſe by the Watch have obſerved,
had it been neceſſarily ſo required ; but the
Parliament never ſaw, or was ever let to
hear or know any Thing of this, or of ſuch
as this, whenas ſuch is or was more material
to be known than all the reſt, as about
which ſo great a Stir was made ; no Trials
of the Performance of my Watch at Sea
needing to be made, or at leaſt no ſuch tedious or troubleſome Trials as were made,
and the Buſineſs as in Conſequence to have
been ſooner got over, could any right Underſtanding been had in the Matter ; or as in
other Words, the Nature of ſuch Mecha-
niſm to have been truly comprehended, and
the Act of Parliament ſo to have permitted
it ; for then, I ſay, no Trials would have
been neceſſary, ſave only ſuch as muſt belong

long to its adjufting; not meaning adjufting by an Adjufting-Plate, as in fuch
Watches as hitherto common, fuch a Thing
as that not having any Thing at all to do in
the Matter; but there are other Things as
pertaining to the Watch here, as well as to
the Pendulum-Clock above, and the which
I have not as yet, viz. as in this other Cafe,
the Ballance, got exactly right, confequently
not fo truly or ftrictly to bear to fuch an
adjufting as what the farther Improvement
which I have fpoken of, will render it capable of doing, as not yet having had proper
Opportunity for it, and that as chiefly becaufe of the Trouble and Hindrance which
the Lunar-Men occafioned me to have;
but Mr. Ludlam [an Univerfity Gentleman]
fays, that I have had Time enough, whenas
it would have been hard to fay whether
there would ever have been Time enough,
viz. to bring, or to have brought, this fmall
Machine, my Watch, to what it is capable
of bearing, and that is to fuch a Truth, as I
myfelf at firft, as well as others, (nay, Mr.
Ludlam himfelf) could think no other, but
to have been—as quite impoffible, [a Second
in a Fortnight] but now I am fure it can be
Matter of Fact. * I fay this might have
been

---

* But as in fuppofing this nice Accomplifhment [or
the Parts from whence this Truth is to be as chiefly
from) not to be truly hit upon in every Watch, but as
in now and then one to be a little wrong, infomuch,
that

been the Cafe, had it not pleafed God that
I have lived fo long; and as ftill to my farther Improvement, I may not perhaps hit it
quite right at the firft, but that fome Experiments may be to be as ftill for a little
Time waited for; * but when once in this,

the

that the Watch may as thence fometimes vary 4 Seconds in a Fortnight, yet ftill, certainly that will be a
doing its Bufinefs well, but if more wide than fo, it
may then be looked upon even as to be done in a care-
lefs Manner, or by a Perfon or Perfons unqualified for
the Purpofe; but perhaps it may withal be fo foolifhly
contrived, or varied in its Conftruction, as to aim at
its coming cheaper, or to be fooner done, whenas, to
have the Longitude to fuch Perfection or Exactnefs,
muft be deferving of any Thing, and as in Confequence
thereof, [v z. of fuch great Safety in the Matter] nothing ought to be wanting, neither confequently any
fuch proper Conveniencies, fo as whereby fuch Watches
or Time-Keepers may the moft certainly be adjufted;
not implying [or meaning at all] the adjufting of fuch
foreign, or nonfenfical Things to the Matter, as about
which fo great a Stir or Noife has been made, neither
of fuch other Imaginations as would ftill be abortive,
although as whence pretending to fhew how far the
Thing may be carried, and that as when moreover, of
notwithftanding, the Sillinefs therein, viz. as pertaining
to the tacking about in a brifk Gale.

* But as thus withal, from the Series of Experiments, which I at laft, through Length of Time, &c.
have been able to make, I can boldly fay or affirm, that
it is fairly demonftrable, [but I think it neither proper
nor neceffary here to fpecify that Demonftration] that
no Time-Keeper, whether in the Pendulum Way, or
in that of the Ballance, can ever be able [through any
Art.ft whatever] to go any higher, or to better mine,
the which, as is fairly to be proved, was far from being
the Cafe with Mr. Graham. Nor could Mr.
Mafkelyne,

the laft Point rightly acquired, may eafily
be done hereafter, and the Watch will perform as I have faid above, viz. fo as never to
deceive the Mariners any Thing material in
their Obfervations, [viz. as when in their
taking the Altitude of the Sun, for finding
the

Maſkelyne, was he to keep my Watch ever fo long,
ever be able to direct how to make it better, no, not fo,
although the firft, and certainly to afford Room for a
much better to be ; but, I fay, was he to fet himfelf
upon fuch a ftrange or foreign Thing, viz. as not only
with Refpect to his Learning, but as withal contrary to
his Bent and Intereft, he could never arrive in the Matter at a *quod erat demonftrandum*, no, neither that it
could be, or not be, as I am now fure, in the Affirm-
atıve, to be the Cafe with me, yea, as furely as that the
Properties of a Circle, and them of Triangles, &c. muft
hold good to Eternity. And indeed it has ever been my
Delight to fearch after, and to come up to Perfection if
poffible, yea, whether I fhould ever have had any Thing
for my Labour or not, and not, I fay, as only bafely or
fneakingly, or as with Uncertainty, to come up with in
the Bounds of the Act of Parliament. And for the which
Perfection, or Safety of Ships, &c. I have indeed had a
long deal of Labour, but, I thank God, I have got it
thorough, whenas no other Purfuit, as rightly to the
Purpofe, will ever be got thorough, and though as with
its having already been a Work in Hand for Ages, yet
ftill, as thence to the Matter, or as notwithftanding
whatever may at any Time be wrote or fchemed about
it, and though ever fo true in itfelf, or in Theory, *I fay*,
ever fo true, yet ftill can but be as upon a bad or dubious
Foundation, viz. as touching any Truth or Certainty
of the Longitude at Sea, and therefore the more there
is of it, and ftill more to be wanted, the worfe as in
Confequence it muft be to be liked, or as thence to be
relied upon.

barely

the Longitude] * and, I think, all ought to
be pleafed, in that it hath fo pleafed God
that I have had fuch Length of Life, &c.
wherein to bring fo noble and ufeful a
Thing to fuch great Perfection, yea, even to
nearly the Truth itfelf ; † but ftill the Profeffors or Priefts as above] muft abfurdly
think, that the Money would be better to
them, than this [or fuch Things as mine]
can be to the Nation, for they wanted fo to
influence the Parliamenr, as to have my
Money, notwithftanding what the Watch
had done ! ‡ And now I am fure, from
my

* But here it may be noted, that what will fometimes render an Obfervation in this Cafe to be 2 or 3
Miles wrong, will or may by the Moon make it as many Degrees wrong, viz. Refraction was parallax, &c.
not to be intermingled.

† But it is to be underftood, that to get fuch a Lon-
gitude-Watch adjufted, viz. to what it will be capable
of bearing, is not to be done [in any reafonable Time]
by one or more of Mr Graham's Clocks, nor indeed
from or by any Obfervation whatever, fave only, as by
or from the Performance of fuch a Clock as mine, confequently any proper Place, or proper Places fo fur-
nifhed, viz. with fuch a Piece or Pieces of Furniture,
muft, where properly wanted, be of very great Utility
indeed , yea, certainly, far to furpafs in Ufefulnefs, or
Highnefs of Ufe, all other Obfervatories in the World.

‡ But what muft thefe men be faid to be done by,
when the Thing was done [viz. fo far as to fulfil the
Act of Parliament] before they began ? and that in the
beft Manner that was, or is in Nature ever to be wifhed
for, out as notwithftanding, would not let it, viz. as in
the

my laſt Improvement, that by or from the Performance of a Watch of ſuch a Size as may be bore with in the Pocket, [but I ſhould not adviſe for it always to be kept there]—the Longitude may be had, and that to a much greater Certainty or Exactneſs, as well as with far more Eaſe and Fre- quency, than ever it will, or can be, by the Moon, conſequently the more by far to be relied upon.

Now, in the former Part of this Book I have treated about Matters pertaining to the Strictneſs of meaſuring Time, and have ſhewn the Deficiencies of ſuch Means as Mr: Graham had taken or made Uſe of for that Purpoſe; and I have alſo treated of the improper, troubleſome, erroneous—tedious Method, which the Profeſſors at Cambridge and Oxford would have to be for the Lon- gitude at Sea : And now I am about to treat of another Concern, the which happened to

F

fall

the whole be paid for, but thought it the more proper to rob the Proprietor of Half his Wages. Whiſton was piſſed on, and Ditton ſhit on, but ſurely theſe Men ought to be beſmear'd or beſpatter'd with both, who, after the Longitude was had by a good and eaſy Way, wanted to have it from a very troubleſome, tedious, difficult, and uncertain endleſs Method! or rather as from uncertain endleſs Methods! For, beſides as from the Moon, from Jupiter's Satellites, the which, as with Reſpect to our needful Purpoſe of Longitude, are not worth mentioning ; but ſtill, or as notwithſtanding, they certainly muſt, by the Hand of Providence, be Highly Created, as well as the Moon, for ſomething elſe ; and therefore they ſhould rather have told us—for what,

+ ſee an addition p. 109

fall in my Way, and the which [at leaſt to
the Royal Society of London, for the Improvement of Natural Knowledge in every
Reſpeƈt] muſt be well worth regarding
when rightly conſidered [at leaſt I think it
ought to be ſo] as being ſo ſecret a Diſcovery; and that is the really true Scale, or
Baſis of Muſick, ſince for which Knowledge, the Muſicians might have played, or
fiddled for ever, and tuned, or have had the
Organ turned wrong in the Church for ever,
and the muſical Part of the Mathematicians
might have reaſoned as they have done, and
wrote about it for ever, and never have
found upon what Foundation the Truth of
the Matter exiſted; and here, as in the firſt
Place, it may not be improper as in particular to remark, 'that Mr. Huggens was, in
his Conjeƈture, a great deal wrong; and my
Friend Dr. Smith [Maſter of Trinity Col-
lege, Cambridge] not knowing that I had
had any Thing to do in the Matter, though
he and I had been pretty intimately ac-
quainted for two Years, and had known
each other much longer, and as Mr. Graham
afterwards told me, that he (the Doƈtor)
had then had his Book, viz. upon this Sub-
jeƈt the Scale of Muſick under Hand for
longer than that time; but as finding reaſon
to think, viz. as from or upon an accidental
Conference which happened betwixt him
and me, that I was in the right, ſaid, that
he would drop his Book, and that I might
make

make the beſt of mine, but inſtead of that,
did ſome Time after, alter (viz. rather perhaps than to loſe his Labour) from what he
had grounded his Work upon, and ſo as to
come as near to me, as he himſelf afterwards
told me Demonſtration would let him, and
then publiſhed it; whenas it is certain, that
if he had not happened to have converſed
with me about the Matter, he had printed
his Book upon his firſt Ground or Principle,
and had then been demonſtratively ſure of
its being right, whenas it was far from
being ſo, though not ſo far as Mr. Huggens's
Conjecture was before him; and it is certain
that neither Theory, Demonſtration, nor
algebraical Reaſoning can have any Thing
to do in the Matter, his own Proceedings
being even a Proof to the contrary, for had
ſuch in the Caſe been Fact, Why did he
alter? or rather, How could he have found
Room or Occaſion to have altered? And as
ſtill farther to remain a little wrong, notwithſtanding his Alteration or Amendment;
and as moreover to expreſs what paſſed betwixt him and me, in his Preface to his
Book, much wrong, inſtead of his being
pleaſed that there was, or is indeed, a firm
and true Foundation of Muſick; but that,
or all this, was not the worſt Jarr that happened betwixt him and me, for, as I could
not adhere to him in the Caſe, he afterwards
turned from being my Friend in the Longitude Affair, to his being therein no better

than

than an Enemy, and perhaps (as already
hinted) in fearing that he fhould through
me lofe his Labour, or that his Book fhould
become of low Efteem, viz. from my Foundation or Difcovery of the Scale of Mufick,
as being indeed the only right one, and
fhould therefore as in Confequence be
ftronger than his;* for indeed, his neither
is, nor can be, any better than as an arbitrary Conclufion, for, as touching Melody,
the chief Matter, it will not afford a Tune,
when ftrictly put in Execution, to any right
or true Content; neither, as touching Harmony, will the fine Chords, the Sharp 6th
and Flat 3ds, rightly bear with his Divifion
or Allotment (this is meaning after his Alteration) whatever he might judge in either
Refpect from mean or falfe Experiments to
the contrary, and his faying as near as Demonftration would let him; the whole Matter [as I have verified, and can at any Time
verify] being as otherwife eftablifhed by
Providence, for I am very fure [and was
then] from the moft ftrict Experience that
can poffibly be made or had, that my Foundation is true, and that it is impoffible
[from the Nature and Nicenefs of the Sub-
ject] for any Thing elfe in the World to
define the Matter; nay, befides myfelf, it
has been allowed or attefted by feveral Mufical Gentlemen, Organifts, &c. who heard
the

---

* So he feemed, as it were, determined to keep me
weak, if he could.

the Refult [of, or upon what it is grounded]
to be in Reality Perfection itfelf, whenas he
[the Doctor] was fo obftinate in the Matter
as not to be prevailed upon—by all the in-
viting, or entreating Speeches that I could
make, to come to hear it! viz. after I had
fufficiently provided for proving the Truth
of the Thing! [viz. more fufficiently than
what I had done from the firft¹] And indeed, the chief Head or Confequence in the
Scale of Mufick, viz. the Intervals of Melody, are, as I may affert them truly fweet,
or mathematically perfect, though never
before were thought to be fo, or that there
was fuch a Field in Nature as wherein they
could be fo, but a foolifh Imagination fure!
Since a good Voice never fails, but can
always, and without any Difficulty, turn
off a Tune, or even a Piece of a Tune, truly,
viz. as without any Regard to the Key, as
hath been foolifhly advanced, and as even
by Dr. Smith could not be; nor indeed
could it be, if the Perfection of the Intervals
of Melody were as the mufical Part of the
Mathematicians have thought they would be
beft, could they be fo had or admitted; as
for Inftance, was the Perfection of the 5th
[as an Interval of Melody] to be as 3 to 2
exact, the Thing [Objection or Suppofition]
would be right, but, as fo, a good Voice
never yet took it, nor never will nor can,
becaufe, if it did, it would be very un-
pleafant, or even ugly, viz. too wide con-

fiderably,

fiderably,* or as more especially to be notified, the 4th to be taken by the Voice, or
by Voices quite out of Tune wide, viz. as
with regard to Harmony, or to the Harmony of 4 to 3 [it not bearing in that Refpect fo much as the 5th] and whenas true
Melody requires it fo to be, and to which
the Voice naturally adheres, yea if it wanted
to take no more than as only the Interval of
one fingle 4th,† and ftill again, as with
Refpect to Harmony [viz. as in that ex-
treme fharp State] to what amazing Finenefs
it is when the fharp 6th [viz. as when alfo
in its refpective propernefs of Latitude fharp]
is founded co-temporaneous with it, as I
can now at any Time, and in each of thefe
Refpects, certify from inftrumental Experience, viz. to any who may be proper to
hear the fame, and as thence confequently
produce a Proof, that there cannot be in the
Scale of Mufick, or that the Voice can
never have any Thing to do with fuch chi-
merical Notes or Intervals, as Tones Major
and

* But then (as in fuppofing that the Cafe) the out-
of-tune Uglinefs or Unpleafantnefs (I am fpeaking as
with Refpect to Melody) would be judged, as according to the common Notion of the World [and that for
Want of accurate Experiments in the Affair] to be as
then, from its not being exactly as 3 to 2, but wider.

† And here it may be notified, That four 4ths and a
fharp 3rd, each in the State nonfenfically ftiled perfect,
will not make two Octaves, no, not by a good deal ;
whenas, four natural 4ths, and a natural fharp 3rd,
both muft and will exactly do it.

and Minor imagined of old; fo the Symmetry therefore as implied, of all the true Intervals of Melody, and as muſt in conſequence thereof be alſo of the moſt rational, or graceful Chords of Harmony, can have nothing to do with ſuch arbitrary Conjectures as have been advanced (viz. as according to Holder's harmonical Nonſenſe in the Affair, ſurfeiting Stuff ſure! though he ſpeaks of it with great Admiration) but are on the contrary, and as I have verified from due Experience, ſecretly grounded upon the true Relation, or as ſtrictly touching this Matter, may be ſaid amazing Proportion which the Diameter and Radius of a Circle bear reſpectively to the Circumference; viz. as thus, As the Diameter and Radius of a Circle bear reſpectively to the Circumference, ſo do the ſharp 3rd, and, as here properly ſpeaking, larger Note bear reſpectively to the Octave (no Tones Major and Minor being in Nature, as of old imagined) and from whence all the others are generated, have you as many Keys, viz. by Flats and Sharps, as you pleaſe,* I ſay, as thence

F 4   in

---

* But here it may be noted, that there can be no Occaſion for ſo many Flats and Sharps in an Organ for a Church, viz any farther than for what Key the Whimſies of the Organiſts may want to play their Voluntaries, &c. in, viz. Things that need not to be played there at all; Time, in Divine Service, being to be otherwiſe employed, and that, as not only more ſuitably, but even as more takingly to the Purpoſe ſo to

be

In the Whole, [and that as from the moſt
ſtrict Experience, viz. as by or from the
moſt ſtrictly due Apparatuſſes to the Purpoſe,] are generated to a mathematical Degree of Sweetneſs, if I may ſo term it, as
well as to be to a ſurprizing mathematical
Degree in Proportion, as being ſeemingly
from a Thing quite foreign to the Matter,
yet ſtill a wonderfully ſtrong, and ſtable
Foundation indeed! But certainly, as the
Works of God are in all Reſpects perfect,
ſo his Praiſe, ſo far as may ever be in Relation

be done: But indeed, a more ſuitable Conſtruction of
the Organ muſt be highly neceſſary, or elſe, a Conſort
of good Pſalm-Singers muſt ever be diſobliged by it, or
not come there, or to where it is at all, ſince their Performances as thence, could but ſeldom be as it were
truly genuine, or naturally
good; ‖ but notwithſtanding
as in, or as with Reſpect to
that Caſe, as ſuch the ſaid
Performances are not as now
to be heard, neither to be
remembered, they, viz. the
Congregations, with the Charity Children, and in their
paltry piece-meal, hodge-podge Manner, can bawl or
ſquawl away along with the Organ, as if ſuch the ſaid
Children were the moſt proper Inſtruments, or Aſſiſt-
ants, for, or to the Purpoſe, and are ſometimes ſet at
ſuch a Pitch, with, or by the Organ (although but
one Part ſung) as to be even fit to ſplit one's Head (an
Abſurdity ſure) yet ſtill I ſay, to be as ſo thought the '
moſt proper, but 'tis not ſo thought to be the Caſe at
the Play-Houſe, viz as with Children there, but certainly, God Almighty never intended that ſuch the
latter ſhould ever excel or over-ſet the former.

‖ And I ſhould have thought
this ought, as ſo highly neceſſary for good Pſalmody in a
Church, to have been Dr.
Smith's Study [as a Parſon]
rather than the Extravagancy
of ſo many Keys.

tion to this [not meaning the Play-Houfe]
muft require to be fo too;* but ftill, fo long
as the Foundation of Mufick lay hid in fecret, unknown of to the World, as alfo the
Knowledge of any fuch nice Preparations or
Ways of proceeding as might or muft be required, in or for its Verification, *i. e.* fo as
whereby to know whether it was or was not,
or might at any Time, really be difcovered
or not, viz. whenever, or if ever that was,
or could be fo deemed as likely to be the
Cafe; but I fay, fo long as it lay hid, the
Confequence was, that it did not feem to
have any abfolute or real Foundation at all;
for, as in the mufical Part of the Mathematicians,

---

* And to which Purpofe it muft be, that in or from
his Completion of Humane Voices, they do not want
as I have fhewn, to take or make Ufe of fuch nonfenfically perfect Intervals as have been fo weakly or foolifhly
imagined, for certainly, any one Note, whenever taken
in any Tune or Leffon of Mufick, and that whether by
the Voice or upon an Inftrument, ought always to be
exactly at the fame Pitch as with Refpect to the reft,
whenas, if fuch Weaknefs, as intimated could take place,
that would not be, nor confequently Mufick to have
any Scale at all; but ftill, for the Sake as it were of
fuch as that, it all along hitherto fo happened, that
Violence, as with Refpect to natural Harmony, was in
fome Meafure put [as thought for the better] to prey
upon Nature in tuning the Organ, &c. And whenas or
as when, what was done for the beft, was with quite a
contrary Drift thereto, the Whole being thereby for the
worfe affected, and that as not in a very fmall Degree,
and yet the great Mr. Handel among the reft [as not
difcovering the Matter] had his Organ and Harpfichord
fo tuned.

ticians, finding in Computation, or in what they called Theory, a Defect of what they denominated a Comma, and to be as a Thing unavoidable in the Matter, they thought that the Beauty, or Perfection of Mufick, muft in fome Meafure be as thereby loft or prevented; whenas, it is through the fame that it is indeed Mufick, and that to Perfection, yea far furpaffing our Imagination, as from the Whole of this Defcription is manifeftly to be perceived, and confequently the World to be but little obliged to Philofophy here, viz. in condemning the Perfection of the Thing, or the Wifdom of God therein; but however, they wanted to cloke that Deficiency [as they thought it to be] as much as they could, as thinking that it was, or muft be always in fome Meafure, nay in great Meafure, fo done by [or that it permitted fo to be done by] or elfe the Thing [fave only as hereafter through Miftake upon the Violin and Violoncello] could not be fo fine or taking as it was, viz. to be cloked by various Diftributions of fuch and fuch Parts of the faid Comma, to fuch and fuch Chords of Harmony, and, as at the fame Time, without knowing what Portion of which, each Chord refpectively, as touching the Matter, would bear; nay thought indeed, that fuch and fuch a Chord as with Refpect to Harmony [not regarding, or notifying what might belong to Melody, altho'

the

the chief] would bear the moſt [or the greateſt Share in that Defect, as was thought to be the Caſe by Dr. Smith, viz. before he converſed with me] whenas the which in Reality [or as on the contrary, under that Suppoſition] will but bear the leaſt. Strange conjecturing ſure! as being in Conſequence without any ſuitable Experience to the Purpoſe! and yet to prevail through Ages! and as moreover, with the reſpective Bearing of the ſharp 3rd, or the Reſult of that as with Reſpect to Melody [or as even to the Deſtruction of Melody] quite the contrary Way, viz. ſharp inſtead of flat! But indeed the moſt Part took it from the reſt for granted, as ſo and ſo to be, viz. without thinking, or properly experiencing the Matters at all; nay indeed to make Experiments, as thoroughly to the Purpoſe, was quite out of the Way or Power of any of them [or of all the Learning or Knowledge heretofore in the World], but to proceed, and though ever ſo far beyond our Reaſon, I do again certify, nay avouch or affirm, and that as without any Notice at all of the feigned Term of a Comma, that the Intervals of Melody [the principal Matter] are from the Circle, &c. as here above advanced, turned off exactly true or ſtrictly perfect, i. e. as without any the leaſt Bearing, Defect or Infringement at all, viz. as with Reſpect to the moſt true, or natural Steps of any Tune; whenas on

the

the contrary, in the taking a few of them
[viz. by a true conftructed Monochord] according to what we fhould think would, or
ought to be perfect [I fay a few of them,
for all cannot fo be] each fuch one in itfelf,
as with Refpect to Melody, will then have
fuch a Bearing, or be fo untrue or out of
Tune, as not to be bore withal, yea fo, befides the utter deftruction of all the reft;
hence if the tuning of an Inftrument, but as
moft to be notified the tuning of an Organ,
be falfe, or varied from the Refult of the
Circle as I have fhewn [as indeed it has hitherto all along been, and that in a pretty
great Degree, excepting through me, as of
late, that fome Tuners have altered] it is not
at leaft fit for a Pfalm-Tune or Anthem;
for I am very fure, that in its differing therefrom it cannot afford a Tune any more or
better than a Viol, &c. otherwife fretted can
do, and that is as nothing to the Purpofe,
viz. in either Anthem, Pfalm, or Song Tune;
but ftill, as without the Proof, Affiftance, or
Application of a perfect Monochord,* viz.
of fuch a one as I have conftructed, and divided upon the true Foundation here fhewn;
or rather as the more eafy, or as the moft
conveniently to be done, viz. as by the
Help

---

* Nay, for this Purpofe or all true Purpofes, there
muft as in the firft Place be two Monochords, in Order
as whence, by proper Means or Trials to prove the
Truth of the String, or of each String.

Help of a proper Set of Forks tuned the moſt ſtrictly to ſuch a Monochord, for by which, the ſaid Forks or each Fork can be tuned to the thouſandth Part of a Note or leſs;* and I think, that by a proper Uſe of Fire, viz. at a proper Diſtance from the Organ, and as thence by Means of a Thermometer near, or not far from the Organ, that the ſame may be kept to the Degree of temperate Heat [viz. to 55] for during ſuch a Time as may be required for Tuning, by the Forks [meaning the ſame to be of a ſufficient large Size for the Purpoſe] all the Pipes included in an Octave, viz. in what is called the Principal; or at leaſt ſo long, as by proper or due Management of the Fire [as from ſtrictly obſerving by the Thermometer] as that ſome of them, as in chief, may be ſo truly tuned, viz. ſo as whence or whereby to be Checks upon ſuch other Proceeding or Proceedings as may be thought neceſſary, or more expedient to the Purpoſe;† but I ſay, that, as without ſomething

---

* Nay, if a Set of Forks ſo tuned, could be properly, or duly ſtruck, how ſweetly would they play a Pſalm-Tune—ſlowly, nay if in two, three, or four Parts, nothing in the World to beat them; a Monochord or Monochords, as under the ſame, or ſuch-like Circumſtances, to be excepted.

† And by the ſaid Forks [viz. of a leſſer Size] the Harpſichord and Spinet can alſo be ſo truly tuned, that ſome Players, as well as others, have ſaid, that they never did hear the Harpſichord, &c. before.

thing in this Way, it muſt be a very difficult
Matter to have it right, or exactly tuned,
yea though what is here above treated of be
the very Voice of Nature, it not being to
be expected, was there nothing elſe in the
Matter, but that Variations, or Falſeneſs,
muſt ariſe or happen in the Proceeding by
5ths, as according to Dr. Smith; but the
Doctor ſays in his Book, that the Voice Part
of an Anthem ought not to be played upon
the Organ, whenas, I ſhould think it the
moſt material, or elſe it muſt be very immaterial to have an Organ in a Church, and
there for a Pſalm-Tune, the which requires
the greateſt Truth of all; but however, be
it as it will, our Organiſts generally there
take Care to blind Imperfections with ſuch
Stuff as does not at all belong to the Matter;
but certainly a Tune ought, as in the firſt
Place, to be diſtinctly a Tune, and conſequently, in a ſpecial Manner, far from ſuch
Nonſenſe as is uſually played before they
begin to ſing, viz. as from whence, but
hardly to be known what Tune they are to
ſing, and therefore it would be much better
if Imperfections did not want blinding, or to
be blinded! But indeed, the Pſalms in general, upon other Accounts [viz. for want of
better Diſcipline than what there is, and in
which Defect the Parſons are much in fault]
are no better than ſmothered, as will fairly
appear when I publiſh the Treatiſe which I
have

have, as more particularly, drawn up about
the Scale and Ufe of Mufick, as therein un-
veiling that Abufe or Obfcurity!* But to
return,

* Viz. If, as according to Royal David's Declara-
tions, as touching his Deliverances, as alfo of them of
the Ifraelites out of Egypt, as well as others the Works
of Almighty God, his Difpenfations, &c and as with
Praifes, &c. thereunto pertaining, as in the Pfalms, be
as ftill to be had in Remembrance or Veneration, and
that as by the Words or Lines of the Pfalms to be [as
now in the New Verfion] right duly handled, and as
therein implying, for the moft Part, by the going on in
Succeffion, with proper Portions or Divifions of each,
or any Pfalm in hand, viz. as when as fo to be done, or
as fo to be permitted by the Parfons, viz. from a fkilful
Delivery of the Clerk [meaning, the fame as then, to be
as fitly chofen for the Purpofe, as if it was for a Play-
Houfe], i. e if their Dignity [viz. that of the Priefts]
will fo admit it, ‖ and whenas
if not, they ought, and as
with a fuitable Grace [or Af-
finity to the Tune, as well
as at the fame Time, by proper Accents, &c. to enhance
the Nature of the Pfalm] to
do it themfelves, but perhaps
they might think it to be as a
Thing almoft repugnant to
their Preaching, but, no
Matter for that, they ought
not to think it fo, but otherwife, and that as truly be-

‖ I fay their Dignity, not
thinking the Clerk to take any
of their Bufinefs from off their
Hands, notwithftanding, finging Men and Boys in Cathe-
drals have Surplices· But as a
Tenor to this, Dr Smith [upon
our difcourfing] faid to me,
that they could fend us Parfons, but where muft we get
good Clerks? And indeed, to
have a good Clerk, muft, in
great Part, be as a Gift of
Providence, whenas the other
is only as it were from Learning

coming thereto, viz. to be, as it were, with lower
Thought—but higher Efteem, confequently without
any the leaft Pride in the Matter, fo that as thence, according to their Drifts [viz the whole facred Drift,
Scope, or Meaning of each Pfalm] as from their Contents, &c. as the which Contents ought indeed to be,
and that as to a full Intelligence, at the Head of each
Pfalm, that fo the fame might, as at leaft with Reafon,

return, Dr. Smith fays, that the Voice-Part
of

vie with the Mufick, and that, as the moft highly becoming fuch, that fame Part of Divine Service, as therein
to do, or rather, as in other Words, as the moft highly
fitting for fuch the higheft Part of the faid Divine Service, and as under the Gofpel's Difpenfation to be
handled, or fo as to
be for the better re-
garded; † no Notes
withal being to be
played [or in anywife
to found] but what
the Voices fing, ex-
cepting the Octave
below the Bafs, no
Repugnancy of tho-
rough Bafs Nonfenfe
to be ufed in Pfalm-
finging. I fpeak from
due Experience,‖ and
if at any Time, any
of the three or four
Notes, the which the
Voices may fome-
times fing, cannot be
reached or touched
upon the Organ, fuch
an Omiffion would be
no Fault at all, be-
caufe the Voices may,

† Not meaning the Lines of the 148th
and 149th Pfalms, nor them of the latter
End of every Verfe of the 136th, to be
given out, neither do we fing the old
148th Tune, nor old 113th, fuch Tunes,
befides feveral others as of old, being
very unfuitable to the Purpofe neither
as farther, do we ufe the 100th Pfalm
Tune for any Pfalm but the 100th,
having Tunes enough to fuit all other
Pfalms, and their Meafures, as in the
New Verfion [and as not over-looking
therein the 96th and 87th, but for which
Pfalms to have fine and fuitable Tunes]
and indeed it is fitting the 100th fhould
have a Tune to itfelf, and none can fuit
it better than its old Tune, viz as when
fung eloquently or laudably, i. e. as when
at a truly right or natural Pitch with
good Strength of Voices in four Parts
rightly adapted. *see addition p 160.*

‖ That being no other, as with Refpect to Pfalmody, and as I have feen
fairly tried by a Company of good
Singers, than as the Devil's Invention,
for they efteemed it as no better, as
being, with Regard to them, a Debar
to any Beauty in the Matter

or can, do fo well without it, or if, inftead of playing
fo many Parts, they touch (at leaft in the Tenor) all
the Notes which Voices fometimes, or in fome Places
ufe, as in their paffing from one Note to another,
i. e. to act or do in that Point as according to Nature,
and as letting the upper Parts to be fung by the Voices
only, and as when in them, for a Verfe or more, and
beft to fuit the Matter, or fubject Matter in Hand [and
as to be inftructed before-hand by the Clerk] the Treble
to be wholly omitted, I fay in this Manner the Thing
would be much better, or they might do or act much
better

of an Anthem ought not to be played
upon

better than to affect the making such a strange confused
noise, so foreign to the Matter, as they always do, and
therefore, as in consequence
of which [or of the whole I
have shewn] not the Subject
to remain, as under Disguise,
a mere Nothing, ‖ but that,
as on the contrary by Custom,
the commendable Matter here
imply'd to be rendered fami-
liar, as the same, (viz. Custom) has done the Badness of
the Play-house. For a Psalm,
when at so low a Degree as
to be taken or handled as Nothing, must be Nothing, and
who can say the Case is now
any better? Well may the
Play-house prevail, or even
the buzzing Things in the
Street! Wherefore I say, if
such as this, or the Contents
of this, be to be regarded
more than a Play, then it is
certain that the Smothering,
as here above signified, will
by my Writing be unveiled.
But if the Case here be not
reasoned aright, then David,
who was a Type of Christ,
must be inferior to a Priest,
for as farther, if Christ in the
Main contradicted David,
[viz. as touching the Sub-
stance of his Psalmody, as
with Respect to Religion]
they could not both be as according to that same Spirit of

‖ Viz As by the taking for
singing [to the Praise and Glory
of God] here and there three
or four Verses, in a nonsenfical
Manner, as to be without any
right Drift or Reason, and as
so, no Matter in what Version,
because, for such a going on,
Dr Brady and Mr Tate need
not to have made a new one,
nor needs any Parish (deficient
in the Matter) ever to chufe
it, but as still to their Shame
keep on, I say as still to their
Shame, for it must be certain
that such a Proceeding can for
the most Part signify nothing,
save only for the making a
Noise, or Sham with the Organ, and as thence putting as
it were a Slur upon David,
just as if a Psalm, though ever
so well handled, must, or
could not be, as with Respect
to a Sermon, nothing! But as
notwithstanding such Imperti-
nency, as with Regard to the
Royal Psalmist, it may perhaps serve [as according to the
paltry Meaning of such a
Drift] to make the Parson to
go up somewhat more brisk or
chearful into the Pulpit, &c.
and as when it cannot be said,
that there is, or can be now,
quite so much Occasion here
for Preaching, as when St Paul,
&c had to convert the World
from such Heathenism as was
grown upon it, and whenas
the Praising of God [that ever-
lasting Gospel] is to hold to
Eternity, and according to St
John, they sing the Song of
Moses in Heaven, as not being
out of Fashion there.

God, which was yesterday, to day, and must be the same
for ever, but as in consequence, if so, the best Way
would

upon the Organ : * But why does he
say

would be to give Religion over ; but ftill, even from Philofophy, God Almighty ought to be praifed, or highly
praifed for his Works [yea, affuredly as from Aftronomy,
ftupendious Works indeed] ; confequently, if David's
Motives and Ways be not fufficient, fo as whereby to
keep up his Praife, there ought as then to be others
taken : But as in fuppofing it to be (as above) reafoned
aright, then, as in confequence of which, was this
higheft Piece of Worfhip, as here advanced, and as
with proper Tunes or Compofitions once to be right
duly performed in Churches [viz. as with more proper,
taking, or fuitable Compofitions, as well as to be more
properly ufed or handled, than as hitherto common in
Churches, viz. as to be there performed by fome proper
Choice of Men of each Parifh, and that as to their Pleafure without any Salaries, yea more to their Pleafure
than running about in the Fields, and as with their
having a proper Loft or Gallery in the Church,—as fuppofing by a Company of about fifty young Men fo fitu-
ated, not but that fome of
them may be married Men, ||
and as to be right duly in-

|| And for which Purpofe,
entire, we had a Loft erected.

ftructed by the Clerk, as I have known, and as whence,
in the Whole, any one of them would almoft have
thought himfelf half dead,
if he could not have got to
the Church, § and as fo, together with fome Boys for the
upper Parts of fuch Compo-
fitions] how wonderfully
ftrange muft it be ! yea even

§ And I am very fure, that
had there been an Organ, and
withal ufed in fuch a Manner
as hitherto ufed in Churches,
it would have been impoffible
in any of our Singers, ever for
that to have been the Cafe

to where unknown, or unaccuftomed thereto, as if they
were Barbarians to it ! The Pfalms not being as only
properly adapted to private Meditation or Contemplation, were they, as now, in that Way to be regarded,
but as, in chief, David made ufe of their Subject Drifts,
and that to the greateft Advantage, in public Singing,
and who can, or dare fay, that there is no Occafion
for any fuch Method, or Courfe, now to be obferved
or taken, as there was in the Royal Pfalmift's Days ?
But

say so? Why, the Reason must be, because
he never found it to be rightly in Tune [or to
agree with what the Voice and Ear wanted it
to be; I am not speaking here about Pitch],
whenas I am very sure it can be so, or may be
so,

But that as on the contrary, the Drifts of the Psalms,
as with Respect to Singing, to lie as under Disguise
above   So now, as in the Whole, ought it not to be
asked or considered, whether it be not a Shame that
these sacred Things should not be more punctually
handled, or better regarded, than what they are as now?
or whether it was not a Shame that David, &c. ever
wrote them at all, viz. as in Behalf of a public Wor-
ship? as the which latter, indeed, seems to be—by the
Parsons, tacitly thought to be the Case, or otherwise,
one would think that better Care would be taken about
them, viz. about such divine or sacred Precepts, yea
even if less Care was to be taken about a Sermon. *see addition p 110*

* Not that I greatly mind what we call an Anthem;
but a Psalm, viz. with its Tune or Composition of
Musick properly adapted (not such Composition as according to Mr Handel's Taste, of or for a Psalm-
Tune) and so to be pitch'd, as that exactly to suit the
Voices, and sung in three or four Parts by a Company
of Singers as above—what a noble Thing it is!   But
it is to be notified, that a little Bit too high or too low
in Pitch, as the 1-8th Part of the larger Note, will
greatly disoblige the Voices [viz. more than one would
imagine]; I speak from the Experience of 20 Years,
and as with proper instrumental Care for Pitching, and
as in the same Time [or long Experience] I strictly
found or confirmed [as in the Time of Divine Service,
or as therein the best to suit] that one Tune required to
be pitched a little flatter or sharper than another, and as
when, without Experience, one would have thought
that the same Pitch might have done right well, nay,
and that any one, the same Tune, required to be pitch'd
a little flatter in the After-noon than in the Fore-noon
But still, it must be allowed that good Voices for

Psalmody

so, viz. if confisting only of such Stops as may be said to be rightly proper for the Purpose; [consequently, not such Stops, or Musick thereon

Psalmody must have the Preference before all other Instruments; but then [and as here exhibited] they must require to be exactly Humour'd; ‖ but that is what the Organ cannot do, save only as in here and there a Tune, and as at now and then a Season to be excepted, and as still with supposing it to be exactly in Tune to itself, or that it would keep so exact thereto as to what it might be set, and that they could also touch or play thereon such Notes, and only such Notes, as the Voices sing, or rather as may, to the greatest Importance or Enhancement, by them be sung; and so, as we had not an Organ, neither to help us, nor to hinder us, ‖ we had not our Tunes pitch'd according to the fixed Notes of an Organ, nor of any other Instrument, but as only from an Instrument whose Pitch might be set exactly to where it was at any Time to be required, and the which [as from properly small Divisions upon it] I noted, as from Experience, to each Tune respectively, § in order that we might not, in the least, ever be disobliged on that Account, viz. by being at all either too flat or too sharp. And here it may be worthy Remark, that an Organist, who was out of Place, came on Purpose to hear our Singing three different Sundays, and attended the Church both Fore-noon and After-noon, and said [or owned] that it was impossible for a Psalm [or the Psalms] to be so well handled by any instrumental Musick whatever, and wondered how the Singers [the which consisted of Plough-men, Shoe-makers, Carpenters, Smiths, Taylors, Weavers, &c and as with some Boys, singing with their Voices small, for the Treble or highest Part, and with only two Boys at full Strength for the

¶ Not knowing how it might be with the Hebrew Musick; nor, perhaps if we did, should we be therewith content

‖ Viz. Not, as in the Ma n, —an Organ instead of a Psalm

§ Note, The Instrument laid, in its Case un ouch'd, save only for just the Time or Times of its using.

Contra-

thereon to be played, as to be even repugnant to the Design or Nature of Pfal-
mody] || but still in-
deed, to have it exactly
so, nothing more nice
in the World! * And
besides, or as without
the Foundation of the
true or perfect Intervals

|| No, such Deficiency,
and as hath been shewn in
more Respects than that,
surely wanting as great a
Regularity, as was instru-
mentally wanted in the
Mensuration of Time for
the Longitude.

of Melody, as here spoken of [and as ought
certainly to be, nay must as in Consequence
be,

Contra-Part, viz. in such Tunes as we used such a
Part] could ever be brought to such Perfection ; for, the
first Time he heard them, and upon the very first Note,
he was quite astonished §
Now I could instance of other
Gentlemen—Strangers to us,
besides this Organist, who
were also taken with our
Singing, but I will only here
mention one, who, after the
Evening Service, was pleased
to give the Singers a Treat,
and that because, neither

§ And here it may be no-
tified, that nothing can be
more handsome than for the
Parson to sing Bass along with
the Singers (and not to sit gaz-
ing about him, as knowing nothing of the Matter), neither
will it hurt or strain his Voice:
As also, here and there a Man
in the Congregation who cannot
so well sing Tenor.

at St Paul's, the King's Chapel Royal, nor at the
Play-House, had he ever heard the like, though he had
oft Times frequented them Places ; and he also ad-
mired the Decency of our Singers, all standing when
singing [facing the Congregation] with their Basses in
the Front, and in the next Pews the Tenors, &c. and
the Trebles up behind ; yea certainly a finer, or a more
graceful Sight, than to see our Gentry at the Play-
House—a Sight never designed by the Dispensation of
Providence, consequently, never [as a Ceremony] for
any pretended Psalmody—there to be sung in Lent.

* Each Interval of Melody requiring, if possible, to
be even to a mathematical Point of Exactness, and

the

be, the chief, or primary Matter], it would
have been a Thing quite impoſſible, as with
Reſpect to Conſonancy, ever to have brought
the reſpective Bearings [as denominated of
the Chords] to ſuch and ſuch their moſt
proper or reſpective Diſtances or Latitudes,
viz. from each ſuch Ratio, as from which
reſpectively they may be ſaid to be generated [or, as unqualified thence to iſſue],
and ſo as whence, not only to become as in
the firſt Place, and as already avouched, true
Intervals of Melody, but alſo, as at the ſame
Time, viz. from each, as it were their then
correſpondent Seaſonings to afford the moſt
lofty, or the moſt elegant Degrees of Harmony ; yea ſo I ſay, as touching this latter
Point, as well as the other, and the which
as otherwiſe would never have been poſſible
ever to have been brought to a true Deci-
ſion ! whenas, from the Circumference, Diameter, and Radius of a Circle, that Matter
is withal undoubtedly, nay I am very ſure
undeniably, decided, the Chords having as
thence, or from their Allotment exactly as
thence, [viz. no one reſpectively to be in
the

the ſame to be from, or accordingly (as I will once
again affirm) to the Reſult of the Circumference, Diameter, and Radius of a Circle, for I am very ſure that
no other Points or Stations will truly afford a Tune , a
moſt ſurprizing, ſtupendious Matter indeed ! Conſequently, ſuch Stops as they call 10ths and 12ths [if tuned
as they denominate perfect] can have nothing to do with
Pſalmody, nor rightly with any Thing, ſave only ſo as
whereby to help the Organiſt to make a vaſt great, con-
fuſed Noſe.

the leaſt Degree either flatter or ſharper than
as ſo allotted] they have, I ſay, as thence,
a much better Reliſh, or a more lofty
Warbling, viz. in Tunes or Leſſons of
Muſick, than if they could be had from
what has been thought would be perfect;
but ſtill, it is to be underſtood, that, to tune
an Organ, &c. only by the Harmony of the
Chords, viz. as without any other Aſſiſtance (and although the common Method
hitherto practiſed) muſt be quite inſufficient
for the Matter of Exactneſs, or as a Beginning at the wrong End of the Work, and
that for want of a more proper Means ſo as
whereby to ſet out the Steps, or to gauge
the Matters more exactly, ſince as thence,
by a good Tuner, and as without ſuch a
proper gauging, all the Chords may ſeemingly be had or obtained to what they ought
to be, and as when at the ſame Time not
the true Intervals of Tune; the Intervals of
Melody being in themſelves much more nice
or delicate than the Conſonances of Harmony! As for Inſtance, the 5th upon an
Inſtrument, may, as a ſingle Conſonance,
be thought to be very fine [nay is indeed
the moſt fine] when there ſet or taken exactly as 3 to 2, although Voices never take
it ſo [nor can ever take it ſo, that being only
a fooliſh Imagination, and quite out of the
Courſe of Nature], and it may be thought
to be good [viz. upon a Spinet, &c.] when
any where taken betwixt that and the flat

Latitude,

Latitude, at which it is as only, or as rightly
to Perfection to be admitted, viz. as with
regard to its mathematical Point, or Points
of Melody; and the same may be said of
all the reft, *i. e.* as ftrictly touching their
flat or fharp Latitudes refpectively, viz. from
what has been thought would be perfect
[could fuch have had their Admittance];
confequently, it muft be the true Intervals
of Tune, or, as in other Words, the true
ftepp'd Paffages among the different Parts of
Melody [though not to be fathomed by our
Reafon] that gives to Harmony its true or
Finenefs of Relifh, yea fo, as well as to
Melody in itfelf, as in a fingle Part Tune,
or Solo;* and as fo, or that that fhould be
the Cafe, what ought therefore, as once
again, to be faid of the Foundation or Ex-
iftence of the natural Notes, or Intervals of
Melody?

* A Meat Pie (as here by the by) will not be good,
truly fweet, or relifhing, without fome Pepper and Salt:
Nay, in a Peal of five Bells, *i e.* where there is but one
5th, it, viz. that 5th, although feemingly under no
Reftriction of being any otherwife than as what we
fhould think would be truly perfect, yet will not be
right truly fweet, unlefs it be no wider, but exactly
according to the Refult of the Circle as above, as I the
moft ftrictly know from Experience, viz. by fuch Means
as by which, indeed, it was right truly to be known,
confequently, as even from thence alone, was there
nothing elfe, a full Proof is had [as was alfo by my
Apparatus, teftified by others as well as by me], viz. of
what wrong Imaginations about the Matter there has
all along been, or prevailed, in the World ! the true
Foundation of Mufick being unknown, but as on the
contrary, divers Opinions and Nonfenfe about it.

Melody? and to what chief Purpofe muft
the fame, as thence, be faid to be? But
Dr. Smith fpeaks of Perfection being in the
Violin and Violoncello, as if upon them
[at Random] the Inconfiftency, as hath been
·fhewn, could be fo truly humoured, as
whereby the Chords and Intervals to be rendered perfect [viz. as accordingly to what
has foolifhly been fo ftyled], whenas, it is
only their Sort of Sound [or, as in Part,
Surge] that is indeed excellent, or even very
excellent, for concealing of Faults in quick
Mufick; a famous Property indeed! And as
when at the fame Time [as without Fretts
duly placed, viz. as according to the Foundation from the Circle as here advanced,
and the farther Confequence of the Truth
of the Strings, as to be acquired therefrom,
and to be corrected, if or when Occafion]
there can be no real Perfection in them, no
humouring to be in the Cafe (excepting as
when, in a long Note, they hear it wrong,
and flip their Finger a little to make it
better) for (as above) it is certain, that [as
well as by the Voice] any one Note whatever, when taken in any Tune, ought always
to be exactly at the fame Pitch as with Refpect to the reft, or elfe (and ftill as above)
no Scale of Mufick at all; and it is not poffible, as purfuant to what has been faid, that
the Fingers can ftop at all the fundry Places
at which they are, or ought at any Time,
to ftop, and efpecially fo, as with Regard to
their

their playing in different Keys, viz. fo neat
hardly as to the 20th Part of an Inch,
whenas to Perfection, much nearer, nay
very much nearer than fo, is, or muft be
required, and as moft efpecially upon the
Violin, where the Strings are but fhort; or
otherwife, and as chiefly touching any Sort
of Pfalmody, as an Anthem, &c. there can
be no fuch Perfection in them as Dr. Smith
feems, from thefe Sort of Inftruments, without Fretts, to maintain;* but even without
any farther to fay, it is certain that there
muft be greater Faults embraced there, than
could be put up with upon the Organ, Harpfichord, or Spinet; a famous Qualification
indeed in them Sort of Inftruments, as here
above

* For fuppofing a Pfalm-Tune [viz. its Tenor and
Bafs] to be played flowly upon them, and never in the
leaft, at any Time, to flip the Finger [or any Finger]
from where at firft ftopp'd down, or pitch'd, what a bad
Piece of Work would be made! For even, without
Fretts, they cannot (as above) right truly fet their Open
Notes as 5ths in Tune, a 5th, as a fingle Confonance,
and chiefly upon them Inftruments, being good any
where, viz. betwixt and including where it is falfely faid
to be perfect, and the flat Latitude at which in Tunes,
or Leffons of Mufick, it only as fo, can be faid to be;
not but that they may fet them truer [viz. the Open
Notes as 5ths] than they can always ftop other Notes
[the Hand having withal fometimes a great Way to
fhift] but I am reafoning about Perfection, and towards
which (the faid Perfection) in Tuning by the Ufe of
Fretts, mathematically placed, and as according to the
Refult of the Circumference, Diameter, &c. of a Circle,
and as thence on Courfe, or as a very material Matter
in the Affair, the true or certain Diftance of the whole
Length

above advanced! And as very furprizing
on the other Hand, what ought there to be
faid

Length of the Strings, viz. from the Nut to the Fore-
fide of the Top of the Bridge, to be, as by a Lath or
Gauge, the moft ftrictly kept
or obferved, ‖ and as together   ‖ Now this is not to be done
with fuch proper Dentings or   by hauling the whole Bridge
fmall Lengthenings refpec-   at once, but as by difcreetly
tively of the btrings into the   jerking or pinching, at the
Nut [in the firft String ex-   Bridge, String by String
cepted] the whole Length of a thick String not being
rightly concerned in founding clofe up to the Nut
[meaning as from the Thicknefs of the Gut, viz. as
without notifying when ftretched, the Wire upon it, as
in a covered String] but that a little Bit of it, from its
Stiffnefs and lying faft in the Notch, will ftill as it were
remain at reft, or not (as again) be fairly concerned in
founding, but, from the Softnefs of the Fingers, that is
not the Cafe at the Fretts; I fay as thus, and as together with Captain Bentinck's Screws; for indeed, without fuch Screws, fuch Experiments upon them Inftruments, as I am here about to fpeak of, could not well be
tried, whenas, as only then, in the making Ufe of the
larger Note, or third Frett from the Nut, the Strings in
the firft Place being made correct [no eafy Matter to be
done by the Muficians, at leaft at prefent, as being as it
were quite foreign to them; but I am ftill treating about
Perfection] a Touch or Trial of the fharp 6th [the
which, as a fingle Confonance, muft be as fharp as the
Ear will permit] as alfo of the 4th [the which muft as
ftill be fharper, or as rather, with Refpect to Confo-
nancy out of Tune, wide or fharp] will greatly rectify,
or decide the Matter, viz. about the Open 5ths, &c.
nay, as not amifs, a Touch of the firft and fourth Strings
with the Bow under the Strings, will, as a fharp 6th,
[Compound of the Octave] as fharp or wide as ever the
Ear will permit—give fome Confirmation to the Whole;
nay fometimes by thefe, a fmall Fault, or Faults in the
Strings, if towards, or near the Nut End, may, when
                                                    fkilled

faid of the infamous or monftrous Divifion,
by the Ufe of Fretts, as now in common
                                        upon

ſkilled in the Matter, be diſcovered ; and even as hence,
it is withal (as farther) ſufficiently proved, that what
Dr. Smith afferts, as touching
the Scale of Muſick, is not
right, ‖ for, in his making
[or ſuppoſing] the 5th to be
wider, and as alſo [on Courſe]
the whole Note (as they call
it) wider, muſt, as in Conſequence, ſpoil the ſharp 6th,
becauſe as thence, it muſt become wider or ſharper than
what it will bear , now, theſe

‖ But indeed, if a Man be
not able, or cannot be as highly
Maſter in this Concern, viz. ſo
as to make, and prove his
Strings to be, right truly in
Order, he cannot make this
[moſt high'y good] Experi
ment, neither others, as belonging to the ſame Purpoſe,
and as alſo to be, in the firſt
Place, as the moſt highly neceffary

are indeed very material Matters, and that beſides the
other Proofs or Truths which the Fretts will afford ;
but ſtill, as overlooking all this, or ſuch as this, [as
indeed, heretofore unknown or unthought of, but that
as on the contrary, being biaſſed or prejudiced, through
falſe or fooliſh Conjectures, viz. as touching what was
done, or might be done] theſe Inſtruments, the Violin
and Violoncello [notwithſtanding Deficiency] were,
and ſtill are ſaid, and as without Fretts, to be perfect ;
whenas it muſt be, that Faults by their Voices are
cloked or concealed. But here it may be proper to notify, that a Viol [viz. with ſix Strings], to any who
may have a Capacity to put it in Order, or can be in-
ſtructed to know what muſt belong to that, and conſequently to keep it ſo, or always to have, or make it ſo,
will then afford [as in itſelf, and as ſo—the King of
Inſtruments] the greateſt Proof of all, of what is the
real Scale of Muſick ! although an Inſtrument, now—
of low Eſteem, nor was it ever worth any Thing at all,
for during all the while—the which it was in vogue ;
but I ſhall not here treat about its Qualifications to the
Purpoſe, for that would be, as here too long . But I
may here notify, or certify, that an Organiſt, who,
upon the hearing me play ſome Tunes upon my Viol,
                                        owned

upon the Guitars? For certainly the Improvement of Screw-work for the Open-Notes, cannot in the leaſt do any thing towards mediating or bettering the Badneſs of the Scale, or Rudeneſs of the Diviſion thereupon uſed! viz. the ſame which was fooliſhly, and for a long Time, uſed upon the Viols and Lutes,* but that there muſt be, as now again, as well as were then for all the while, —infamous Maſters indeed, viz. for the greatly abuſing of Muſick; for now, from the pretty Voice of the Guitar, viz. in its clokeing ſuch Stuff as can have nothing to do in the Matter, no, far from it, and though in that Point (viz. Clokeing) much better than the Viol, &c. could do, yet ſtill as with Reſpect to Muſick (viz. in the Condition intimated) there can but be as it were a fine Sort of Janglement turned off, for, was a Pſalm-Tune or an Anthem to be played upon it [be ſuch to be notified] the Beauty of Holineſs [as according to the Royal Pſalmiſt] muſt, in the praiſing of God that Way, be very much defaced, true Melody and Harmony being—both as thence ſacrificed, viz. to the Abſurdity from, or by which

owned that it ſpoke to Perfection itſelf; and whenas, without a Monochord, a Spinet or Harpſichord can give no ſuch Proof to the Matter, viz. of what is the true, or real Scale of Muſick—as the Viol in itſelf can do

* Viz. The Octave into twelve equal Parts; two of which to the whole Note, and one to the Half,

which the Fretts are placed; and yet to
this, Ladies of Quality muſt ſing! But what
muſt they ſing? Why, a Shame to themſelves and their Maſters! becauſe it can play
nothing elſe!—But now to proceed, [the
laſt Piece as here above treated, viz. as about
the Guitar, being as it were almoſt a Digreſ-
ſion, and but hardly worthy Notice, but I
ſay,] it ought certainly, as in a high Degree,
to be remarked, that Dr. Smith's Endea-
vours, whereby to find the Bearings of each
Chord, viz. by the Number of Beats reſpectively in any given Time, and as thence to
tune the Organ exactly—could be nothing,
but were pretty much a-kin to the finding
the Longitude by the Moon,* for, as nothing to the Purpoſe could be had that Way,
ſo, in his tuning an Organ, Harpſichord or
Spinet, and as not being on the other Hand
by an accurate Monochord, founded, upon
what he calls his own Principle, neither as
upon that of mine, how could he tell what
was done, viz. as touching any Strictneſs or
Truth in either of them? † But as notwithſtanding,

---

* Now here it may be proper to notify, that no Beat-
ings are to be heard from a Viol when truly fretted, or
rightly in Order, no, nor, if you pleaſe, from two Viols,
playing ſlowly a Pſalm-Tune and its Baſs, viz. any
more, or no more, than as from human Voices, but
indeed, not ſo the Caſe with an Organ, neither with
Muſical Forks, but ſtill, not to be enumerated.

† But a Monochord to Perfection, to have been produced from Cambridge Education, would have been another Thing [viz. ſomething very extraordinary indeed].

ſtanding, whatever Univerſity Men write or
do, it muſt be had in Veneration, as was
the Caſe with Mr. Huggens's Diviſion as
touching the Scale of Muſick;* viz. the
Octave into thirty-one equal Parts, whereof
five of which was to go to what they call
the whole Note, and three to what they call
the half Note Major, whenas, if an Organ
Harpſichord, or Spinet, was to be tuned
exactly thereto, viz. by a Monochord well
executed, and truly divided or ſet off upon
that Principle, i. e. each Diviſion to be
thereupon true to its Place, at leaſt to the
200th Part of ¼ Inch, as ought to be the Caſe
with a Monochord, nay, muſt to the Purpoſe be ſo upon my Principle [viz. as ſet off
with great Accuracy from Logarithmical
Calculations, and as then together with ſuch
a String as muſt ſtill to the Purpoſe be required;† or was a Viol, &c. to be fretted
accordingly as here ſignified, viz. to what
Mr.

* As likewiſe in his Cycloid, viz. as with Reſpect
to any Application of ſuch his Demonſtration to the
Pendulum of a Clock, and where it (the ſaid Pendulum)
muſt move in the Medium of Air, and where, conſequently, the Draught of the Wheels of a Clock muſt
be concerned, and whenas, even without that [or theſe
Matters] it could not, for other Reaſons which I have
given, be as there—for any Good applied.

† For here I muſt notify, or rather certify, that none
of the common Wire '[viz. of the Spinet Wire, &c.]
will do for the String of a Monochord. No. A String
for a Monochord is indeed ſomething very extraordinary,
and

Mr. Huggens thought muſt be the beſt, they would, viz. any, or each of them re-ſpectively, be very confuſedly out of Tune, viz. more ſo by far than what Dr Smith had imagined, and as farther upon his own Conjectures had made, as he thought, very accurate Experiments about; and, as with Reſpect to his Book, no Doubt but that Algebra was made a Tool of, or rather (as in its having nothing to do in the Matter) a Fool of, viz. before he took Occaſion, through his converſing with me, to alter from what he thought he had aſcertained, not meaning that he altered from the Alge-bra, but only in the Algebra, ſo as the better to ſuit with me; but ſtill, as to his Expe-rience or Application thereof to an Inſtru-ment (as already ſhewn) there could be no Proof, either of his Principle or mine, or rather, as in other Words, no Proof at all of what he had brought his Principle to, as in Compariſon, or Conſequence of mine! And yet to publiſh upon ſuch a ſilly, weak Foundation,

and of very great Moment, and that as unknown to the World before ! But I ſhall not here treat of its Proper-ties or Faculties; but however, it is very practicable to be produced, ſince as now, after my Diſcovery of ſuch unimagined Secrets or Faults as would pertain thereto, and as not only ſo, but alſo how to prevent the ſame, and render the Matter perfect, it is no great Difficulty to be had [but ſtill, not that every one will do] as is to be verihed from divers Sorts of Experiments by two Mo-nochords, truly perfect in other Reſpects, the old No-tions of a Monochord being even as nothing at all towards the Matter.

Foundation, or infufficient, uncertain Way
of trying, as wherein (for ought he could
prove or affure to the contrary) mine might
be taken or aimed at, inftead of what he
calls his own ! O fie ! Infamous Cambridge
Craft indeed ! Such Experience as that, not
being able to verify the Truth of what he
thought, or might think, he had brought
the Alteration of his Book to ! * for, from
his converfing with me, be his Book what
it will, or whether it had ever been wrote
at all or not, or even whether he had ever fo
much as thought about it at all or not, he
might, from that Way to work, have done
the very fame ! Univerfity's Ingenuity ! Nor
can any the beft Player upon the Violin, &c,
[viz. as without Freſts, or any adjufting, or
correcting of the Strings as whence to be
verified] ever as thence know what is the
real Scale of Mufick ; for fuppofing he could
ftop, or may ftop exactly to, or in fuch
Places as at which his Ear may beft like it,
or even, as exactly to what he ought to
ftop , yet I fay, as thence, he can have no
Mathematical Account of the Proportions or
Intervals of the Scale, or of what is the Scale

H

of

---

* But Dr Smith fays, that he directed Mr, Turner,
an Organift, fo as to put his Way of Tuning in Execution, and that he [viz. Mr. Turner] approved of it
very much But here, it muft certainly be worthy Remark, that it had never been the Doctor's Way, had it
not been mine firft

of Mufick he makes Ufe of: As for Inftance, No one, even any the beft Player, could ever tell whether he played the fharp 3rd exactly to what is faid would be perfect, or whether he played it, as with Refpect thereto, a little flat or fharp, in Order that it really fhould be fo; no, no more than what a good Singer as by Nature can, and that is as thence or thereby—none at all; confequently, fuch a Performance can have nothing to do with the Application of the real Scale of Mufick to the tuning the Organ, Harpfichord, or Spinet. Now, Mr. Graham never fo much as offered to befet, befpatter, or befiege my Proceedings, after any fuch Rate or Manner; but, as notwithftanding, Mr. Ludlam could: But now, upon my firft telling Mr. Graham that the Doctor and I could not chime in right about the Scale of Mufick, and that I believed I had loft a good Friend as with Refpect to the Longitude Affair, he [viz. Mr. Graham] was very much difpleafed, and thought that, inftead of the Doctor ufing me ill [viz. as by his taking or letting the Accuracy of my Labour as nothing] he ought, as an upright, ingenuous Man, to have been pleafed that Mufick had fo good a Foundation, and fo as to put an End to all Difputes and Conjectures about the Matter, and Lord Macclesfield alfo expreffed the fame; however, I kept to my Integrity, not minding the Lofs of a Friend, and who

I

I had fo great an Efteem for, and would
very gladly have had him to have taken the
Matter [as in its true Light] quite off my
Hands [viz. before he publifhed his Book,
or as even from the firft Time that we con-
verfed about it] as thinking he had both
more Time and Art than I, viz. fo as
whereby the more handfomely to communicate both it and it's Ufe to the World;
but that he would not do, as pretending
[viz. after he had altered his Book] that
Demonftration would not let him, the which,
as I have fhewn, could be nothing; but as
I was certainly in the right, and ftanding to
my Integrity I loft his Friendfhip, and indeed it was with Tears;* but this is the
Way of the Univerfity-Men, they want to
fuck the Virtue out of every Body's Works,
and then to call all their own; for through
me, he [the Doctor] brought his Scale of
Mufick very near to mine, or nearly to the
Truth, but, as in the Main to be taken,
left a little Difference, that it might be called
his, and not mine: Nay, with Refpect to
thefe Sort of Men [or Univerfity Gentlemen]
I have fmelled a Defign, of the fame Sort or
Kind, upon another Difcovery of mine—
befides this, and that a fecret as this; and
the which had never been difcovered at all,

had

* Not that he had any great Skill in the Matter
[viz. of my Machinery] but did me good, nay a great
deal of good, from what Mr. Graham faid of it.

had it not been through some Transactions
I had with my third Machine; consequently
as so, and as to be so very weighty, or so
highly useful a Matter or Discovery as it
was, and as never to have been known or
discovered without it, it was therefore Longitude enough for it, and worth all the
Money and Time it cost (nay, it was even
withal, as some Requital towards the Loss
or Expence of the other two) viz. my curious
third Machine; and the which, with the
other two large Machines, was the most
scandalously sacrificed, viz. by a Novice, as
at, or to his Pleasure employed—by the
Board of Longitude.

Now, Mr. Graham allowed that his Methods for a nice Mensuration of Time, were
insufficient as with Respect to mine; but
that was far from being the Case with Dr.
Smith; he was a Parson, and they are
strange Things!

And now I think, that the drawing up of
this Book, and as together with the Drawings and other Writings I shall leave [and
especially them of late] as illustrating why
Time-keeping can indeed be so truly had,
must, if their Virtue can be kindly received
---be better to the Public than if I had finished or completed ten Longitude Time-
Keepers; no (Lord Morton's) Chance to
take Place in my Proceedings: For, towards
a Proof of which, let it be remembered, that

I

I have said in this Book, that if it pleased
God to continue my Life and Health a little
longer, that then, from my laſt Improvement, I would bring my Watch or Time-
Keeper ſo as to perform to a Second in a
Fortnight ; and now, ſince the drawing up
of that Part of the Book, I have indeed put
the major Part, but ſtill not the moſt nice
Part thereof, viz. of my laſt Improvement,
in execution, not venturing, upon ſerious
Thought, to attempt the Whole, leſt I
ſhould not live to ſee it perfected, and I now
find the Watch to perform as above ex-
preſſed, nay even to nearer than ſo ! but
ſtill no aſtoniſhing Matter, ſave only to
them [or ſuch Philoſophers] who cannot be
able to weigh its Conſtruction, or the main
Points of its Contrivance, and as wherein
hardly to be influenced, whether any Oil or
not : But indeed, had I continued under the
Hands of the rude Commiſſioners, this
Completion, or great Accompliſhment, neither would, nor could, ever have been obtained ; but however, Providence otherwiſe
ordered the Matter, and I can now boldly
ſay, that if the Proviſion for Heat and Cold
could properly be in the Balance itſelf, as it
is in my Pendulum, the Watch [or my Longitude Time-Keeper] would then perform
to a few Seconds in a Year, yea, to ſuch
Perfection now are imaginary Impoſſibilities
conquered ; ſo the Prieſts at Cambridge and
Oxford,

Oxford, &c. may ceafe their Purfuit in the Longitude Affair, and as otherwife then to occupy their Time.

I will now give fome Account how the real Scale of Mufick is indeed generated from the Proportion which the Diameter and Radius of a Circle bear refpectively to the Circumference; but, as towards which, this great, or fecret Difcovery, it is, as in the firft Place, to be underftood, that it was after I had made feveral ftrict Experiments of divers, or diverfe Divifions of the Octave, and they as from or by fuch neceffary, or proper Preparations, or Aparatuffes to the Purpofe, as from my other Bufinefs I was enabled to make; yea, I may boldly fay as thence, from far more correct, or natural Qualifications to the Purpofe, than any before me were ever able to make or have [nay, and ftill are—as yet the fame], and that, as fo at laft, I found to my great Surprize, or Admiration [viz. as from the fame Strictnefs of Trial of the Refult of the Properties of a Circle, as here above fpecified, and as with fuch, the fame Apparatuffes to the Purpofe] the real Foundation of the Matter to exift, or to be, as thence, by the Hand of Providence eftablifhed; and the which (as in brief) I fhall explain as followeth.

Let the Ratio of the Octave, or, as even here, as well as below to the Purpofe, the
Octave

Octave itfelf, be reprefented by the Logarithm of 2 [viz. by ,30103]; and let that
fame Number be alfo taken or
fuppofed as the Circumference of
a Circle   -   -   -   ,30103

And then [as in the Margin]   2
let the Space or Quantity of two   —————
Octaves and a fharp 3rd be taken,   ,60206
or be as chiefly, or rather as pri-   ,09582
marily to the Purpofe notified,   —————
viz. when [as according to my   ,69788
Difcovery] the faid fharp 3rd is in   —————
its moft ftrictly mufical Propor-
tion, and that is as when, with Refpect to
the Octave, the fame is taken as the Diameter of the Circle [viz. here, as ,09582] :
For the Proportion which the Circumference
of a Circle bears to the Diameter (and as
true enough to this Purpofe, as well as to
others) is about as 3,1416 to 1 : So, as
3,1416 is to 1, fo is ,30103 to ,09582.

And then, as five larger Notes [but not
with Tones Major and Minor, as hath been
imagined, and that from of old] and as together with two of the leffer Notes [as all
along foolifhly ftyled half Notes Major] are,
or muft be, exactly contained in the Octave :
So therefore, as in taking Half the Diameter
for the larger Note, viz. ,04791, as I from
ftrict, or proper Experience, found it to be
—as an Interval of Melody, right truly pleafant [although, as barely in itfelf, as well as
the leffer Note, nothing to do with Har-
mony],

mony], and that four 5ths, thence as below
to be generated [viz. of each containing
,17447], and as when, as I am Proof fure,
to be then in their moft ftrictly
mufical Proportion, will, as ac-   ,17447
cording to Nature, be equal to the   4
two Octaves and fharp 3rd; and at   ————
the fame Time, as already inti-   ,69788
mated, each one of the four 5ths
will alfo be as without any Infringement in
any Cafe [viz. as with Refpect to the Product of Nature] fo generated by fubftracting
five Times the Radius from the Circumference, where will be left fuch a Quantity
or Space, as the two leffer Notes muft, with
equal Shares, take up; and that will be
,06148, fo the Half of which, viz. ,03074,
muft be the leffer Note ; and the leffer Note
fubftracted from the greater will leave
,01717, properly to be called a Flat or a
Sharp [or the Difference of the Notes], and
not nonfenfically the Half-Note Minor; the
leffer Note having withal the fame Autho-
rity to be called a whole Note as what the
other has; but they may refpectively or
properly be ftyled Tone Major and Tone
Minor, viz. without meaning the fictitious
Nonfenfe as of old; and (as well underftood) a 5th muft contain three of the larger
Notes and one of the leffer [viz. as in the
Cafe or Cafes here, ,17447].

But as notwithftanding, that from what
'tis here above, are indeed the real Steps or
Th...   Intervals

Intervals of Tune, or of natural Melody,
exactly pointed out, or are to be as thence
truly generated [viz. accordingly as they are
taken by the Voice or by Voices]; fo there
muft, as in Confequence thereof, be alfo the
real Confonances, or Chords of natural Harmony, truly limited or defcribed; nay as
fo, in both Refpects [viz. as touching both
Melody and Harmony] I found, to my
great Surprize, to be confirmed upon ftrict
Inftrumental Mufick, as I have fhewn above.

But ftill (and as juft has been intimated)
that though from what is fhewn above, the
true Steps of Melody, as alfo the true Confonances of natural Harmony, are, as touching them all, or each of them, exactly to
be defined, yet, as from thence, no Ratios
at all can be faid to be (that of the Octave
to be excepted), fo the faid Chords, &c.
muft be denominated as they have all along
been; and, in the Logarithm Way, as here
to the Purpofe the beft Way, as the Ratio
of any Chord is to be had by fubftracting
the Logarithm of the leffer Number from
that of the greater, fo therefore, and as only
proper, viz. as in what is here, as firft above
—may differ from fuch Ratios, fo each
Chord, or Interval, muft to its Propernefs,
or Sweetnefs of Relifh, in Tunes or Leffons
of Mufick, be faid to have refpectively fuch
and fuch Flatnefs or Sharpnefs of Latitude;
as the 5th to have ,00162 flat Latitude, the
4th (its Complement to the Octave) as much

I   fharp;

sharp; the sharp 3rd to have ,00109 flat
Latitude, the flat 6th as much sharp; the
flat 3rd to have ,00053 flat Latitude, the
sharp 6th as much sharp; and here I may
notify, that the 3^{rds} will bear their flat Latitudes better than the 6^{ths} will bear their
sharp; nay, the 5th will bear its flat Latitude of ,00162 as well or better than the
sharp 6th its sharp Latitude of ,00053: But,
to bear have I said, as touching them all!
whenas, as when in that, their exactly right
Degrees, they are only as so rendered perfect! I speak from strictly due Experience
[viz from such as no Man before me could
ever make, nay, and are as still the same];
and therefore, as each Interval respectively
so results from the Properties of a Circle, as
I have shewn, they cannot each one, or any
one, as by a Proof from thence, be said to
have a Defect of any Part or Parts of a
foolishly feigned nonsensical Comma; nor
for this, as here otherwise shewn, is certainly
the true Essence of all that can be said of
the Matter, whatever Nonsense any Book,
as heretofore in the World, may consist of.

Now, whether my Style of Writing in
this Affair, be right proper to the Purpose
or not, I thought it must be better than
that the Contents of this Book should be in
Danger of sleeping in Oblivion; yea, notwithstanding what I had—as verbally communicated to the World.

FINIS.

APPENDIX.

LET the following Addition be joined to the End of the Note on Page 43, viz. after the Words *put or infused Chance into their Heads:*—But, as here to return, Mr. Shepherd thought it ftrange that he could not be made able to comprehend my Watch, as well as (he exprest it) Jonne Ludlam.

In the Note on Page 67, after the Words, *as with Refpect to our needful Purpofe of Longitude, are not worth mentioning;* let this Interline, as here following, be taken; —for even at Land, an Obfervation therefrom may, perhaps, fometimes be 4 Minutes from the Truth, as fo happening from their acting one upon another;—but ftill, or

K   Let

Let what is here following be joined to
the fecondary Note on Page 82, viz. after
the Words *with good Strength of Voices—
in four Parts rightly adapted.*—And here it
may be worthy Notice, that (in any Pfalm)
as a Grace to the Matter, the Trebles and
Baffes, at the End, or laft Note of each
Line, do continue to found a little after the
Tenors and Counter-Tenors have done, but
the Baffes, of the two, rather the longeft;
and as thus, with the chief Matter, viz. as
with the Lines [or Words] given out as in
a proper, intelligent Manner, the Subject
is, or muft be as thereby, very much fet off
or 'enhanc'd, and as whence withal the
Singers have Refpites for their Voices; and
certainly, as fo in the Whole, the Matter is
or becomes very taking and good, or, as
according to St Paul, very rich; but the
Parfons take but little Care about this Sort
of Richnefs, but for the moft Part to render
it Poornefs, confequently as fo, or as whereby to become no fmall Contributors towards
the upholding of the Play-Houfe; and at
which Rate the Devil's Glofs that is upon
the Play-Houfe, muft excel or outweigh the
Divine Stamp that is upon the Pfalms.

And let this following be joined to the
Note on Page 85, viz. after the Words,
if lefs Care was to be taken about a Sermon;
                                        —for

—for even in this Point it is withal, from their Careleffnefs, to be obferved, viz. the wrong Tranfmutation in fome Places of the Pfalms [as in fome Books or Impreffions without Authority] fince Tate and Brady left 'em. But here, it is as farther to be notify'd, that an Organift who plays in the Church, may or can alfo play in the Play-Houfe; as alfo any Girl, who, as they think, fings fine in the Church [though even there as nothing in Comparifon to what Church Singing ought to be] may alfo fing in the Play-Houfe; but then, ought it not to be afked, Why does not the Clerk, &c. at the Church, or of the Pfalmody there, go alfo to the Play-Houfe?—See Bedford's Abufe of Mufick: and whenas his Sentiments about the Matter are not all accordingly to what they ought to be.

SINCE

SINCE the publishing of this Book, a Monthly Review (for October 1775) was prefented to me, wherein I found a great deal of Rancour, yea, even to a high Degree, againft me, but my Anfwer to the Matter fhall be but fhort.

As firft, Let the Profeffors, Commiffioners for the Longitude, come and fhew me whatever Ufe there has as yet been made, or can ever be made, for any good Purpofe at Sea, in the numerous Columns, the which I fpoke of in their Nautical Almanac.

And fecondly, as touching the Scale of Mufick, As they have (in the fame Review) faid, that it is confeffed [meaning by all] that was there but only one Key to be ufed, all its 8 Notes fhould then be tuned perfect Confonances, according to the Diatonick Scale, and as only wherein, a Tune to be play'd perfect, whenas, in what they therein think,---that could not be a foolifh Imagination as of old, even that there ever was fuch a Scale at all, for no fuch Thing is in Nature to be found, but what will have Clafhes in it, and they very great ones too! Whenas certainly, the real Scale of Mufick, when fo far exhibited, as in proper Divifions neceffry, muft afford a Tune, moft truly fweet in itfelf, in any Key, in which, as fo, they

they may be pleas'd to play it, as is the Cafe
in my Difcovery; but they have faid (in the
faid Review) that my Scale only did, as it
were, accidentally fall in with Dr. Smith's
Syftem nearly, whenas Dr. Smith's was
vaftly wide from mine, before he had con-
verfed with me, and altered his! Now
thefe Expreffions are vaftly different *; nor
can it yet be proved, nor ever will, that
Dr. Smith, as without a proper Apparatus,
or rather as without proper Apparatuffes,
could, as at his Pleafure, in tuning the Spinet
or Harpfichord, could [I fay as fo] exactly
tune either to his arbitrary Scale, or to
what is built upon my affuredly true Foundation: And now, if I have written wrong,
as in there not being what they would call a
Diatonick Scale, let them come and prove
that †, and I will not only bear their Ex-
pences, but will alfo pay them for their
Labour.

---

* But ftill, they agree, as well as what is in Dr.
Smith's Preface does, to the Words which paffed betwixt the Doctor and me. Defperate Prieftcraft fure!

† Neither were there ever any fuch nonfenfical
Things, as Chromatick and Enharmonick Scales, as
being [all three] but only fuch imaginary Suff as was
through Ignorance blaz'd, or buzz'd about in the
World, and that to no good Purpofe at all, but mere
Confufion! There being but one true Scale of Mufick,
and that a very ftupendiously natural one indeed! Stu-
pend.ous, I fay, confidering upon what the fame is
grounded, or as from whence the fame to exift!

Labour. Therefore, to conclude, shall write no farther about such Nonsense, Spite and Poison [scandalously scurvy, dirty Work indeed] as runs throughout the Whole of their maliciously groundless Objections, as objecting against Things which are really true and done! Famous Fellows indeed! The like not being elsewhere to be found; the Longitude not being to be right truly proved or completed, so long as such——the said Fellows do reign.

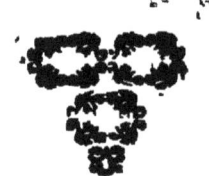

ERRATA.

Page 17. Note, 3d Line, inſtead of *laſt above,* read Page 12.

Page 28. Note, 9th Line from the Bottom, inſtead of *ſpeakingly,* read *ſneakingly.*

Page 65. Note, 17th Line from the Bottom, inſtead of *baſely,* read *burſly.*